# Invisible

# Invisible

HOW YOUNG
WOMEN WITH
SERIOUS
HEALTH ISSUES
NAVIGATE WORK,
RELATIONSHIPS,
AND THE
PRESSURE TO
SEEM JUST FINE

## Michele Lent Hirsch

BEACON PRESS
BOSTON

BEACON PRESS
Boston, Massachusetts
www.beacon.org

Beacon Press books
are published under the auspices of
the Unitarian Universalist Association of Congregations.

22 21 20 19     8 7 6 5 4 3 2

This book is printed on acid-free paper that meets the uncoated paper
ANSI/NISO specifications for permanence as revised in 1992.

Text design and composition by Kim Arney

This is a work of nonfiction. The events portrayed are presented to
the best of the author's memory and records.

Many names and other identifying characteristics of people mentioned
in this work have been changed to protect their identities.

*Library of Congress Cataloging-in-Publication Data*

Names: Hirsch, Michele Lent, author.
Title: Invisible : how young women with serious health issues navigate work,
    relationships, and the pressure to seem just fine / Michele Lent Hirsch.
Description: Boston : Beacon Press, [2018] | Includes bibliographical
    references and index.
Identifiers: LCCN 2017026791 (print) | LCCN 2017054082 (ebook) |
    ISBN 9780807023969 (e-book) | ISBN 9780807029817 (pbk. : acid-free paper)
Subjects: LCSH: Sick—United States—Social conditions. | Women—United
    States—Social conditions. | Sick—United States—Psychology. |
    Women—United States—Psychology.
Classification: LCC RA418.3.U6 (ebook) | LCC RA418.3.U6 .H57 2018 (print) |
    DDC 305.9/0870820973—dc23
LC record available at https://lccn.loc.gov/2017026791

*For Simon,*
*even after all the changes*

# CONTENTS

# AUTHOR'S NOTE

When a fistful of serious health issues struck me in my twenties, I saw how being young and female was inextricably linked to my experience. That I looked bright-eyed and "feminine" affected how others responded to me, too. Often, people thought that I looked *great!* or *pretty!* or *young!* and that I therefore couldn't possibly be sick. So I began to interview other young women who'd been through a lot. And I saw that for each person I met, words carried their own meaning.

Language is a tricky thing, especially when we try to capture what's happening in our bodies and in our culture. Words like "health," "healthy," "sick," "illness," and "disability" are always relative and always loaded, rarely static, and often problematic. Words like "women," too. Our definitions are constantly in flux—as are, for instance, the laws that govern our rights. Whose bodies count? Whose bodies do we systematically inconvenience or overlook? In this book, I've tried to be mindful of the fact that a phrase that resonates with one person may feel prickly, even hurtful, to another. Some women I've met identified as having a health issue, some as having a disability. Some spoke of how their sexuality, gender identity, or race intersects with their experience, while other women—often those who face less discrimination or who have more privilege—didn't bring up those aspects of identity nearly as much.

I'm also aware that one small book trying to start a big conversation can't possibly discuss every type of health issue out there.

Nor have I captured a perfect cross-section of women. That said, by trying to interview women from different backgrounds—whether in terms of gender identity, race, sexuality, geography, economic status, or beliefs—I hope to sketch a picture of what it's like to be young, female-identified, and dealing with the constant pressure to seem youthful and carefree, no matter what one's body is going through.

# PART 1

# Could Someone Love
# This Body of Mine

*He must see my scar*, I think, but the bar is dimly lit, as bars are, and for the first time I understand the lighting. The back room that I had to shimmy through a crowd to get to is hopefully dark enough to hide the red slash across my neck. Hopefully.

The guy in question is asking about the vintage pin on my coat. I AM A TRAINEE PLEASE BE PATIENT, it reads. Mustard yellow, all caps, no punctuation.

"Oh yeah, I got it at a thrift shop, sort of a fancy junk shop," I tell him. "Probably some person in 1972 was miserable when they had to wear it while training for, I dunno, a cashier job or something, and now I'm the jerk who misappropriated it years later and stuck it on my jacket to be hip."

"I'm Simon," he says. He seems amused by my self-deprecating answer. I don't mention the part about how the pin doubles as an existential joke, some cheesy thing about how we're all just trainees. Simon seems to get it. I don't mention, either, the hope flickering in my head that people I meet will be patient with my body.

We talk for an hour at first. Simon is charming, an unexpected highlight after a bookstore reading I'd gone to with a coworker. The friends he'd been at the bar with and my friend from work wave to us, comically wink at us, but it doesn't register. We talk for four more hours until, at some point, we realize how late it is, that everyone else has left. Then, finally, we kiss.

On our first official date a few days later, Simon asks about my neck. "What's that scar from? Is it new?"

"Uhh . . . you should have seen the other guy," I say, which is ridiculous, really, because I despise when people say that. I despise that phrase in particular and I despise clichéd euphemistic cover-ups in general, but I say it anyway. I'm not going to tell this sort-of stranger that I look like a regular chick and all but actually just had my thyroid cut out. That the cancer had spread from a butterfly-shaped organ we forget helps keep us alive and asserted itself in several of my lymph nodes. That in a few weeks I'll need radioactive treatment to kill the remaining cancer cells that might be swimming in my neck. Or that I'll be quarantined during the treatment, a biohazard. No way.

*Once you have a health problem, it's over.* It's a comment I both recall hearing and yet can't pin down: a woman, or an amalgam of women, in person, on television, warning me that what happened to her will happen to me. Women who told me about the men who left them, who couldn't handle illness or just didn't want to or—what's the difference? Young acquaintances whose partners got squeamish the moment health issues came up. Older friends, too, with resigned looks on their faces as they remembered their early twenties. The decades they've spent dealing with their health and then, on top of it, with lovers who ran away.

But when I became that twentysomething with an array of medical issues (hip surgery, mast-cell activation syndrome, Lyme disease, thyroid cancer—an improbable series of health crises that swiftly changed my idea of youth), I realized how many young women deal with the same. And because my father, who'd had multiple sclerosis, ended his life in the midst of my own health experiences, I became even more aware of the ways that different people react to their bodies. Unlike my father, though, I wanted very much to live.

So I began to gather stories. I learned how women from across the country dealt with no longer feeling invincible like their young peers. How they feared being rejected if they mentioned their health issues. How that fear often motivated them to hide the ways their bodies worked. I heard about the actual rejections they'd experienced, in the workplace and in social settings, and how our culture led them to expect the worst even from partners and bosses and friends who seemed to wholeheartedly accept them. How gender norms and the idea of "perfect" young bodies played out in both queer and heterosexual relationships, and how the specter of feeling like a freak hovered above them differently.

In a 2012 study from the journal *Qualitative Social Work*, researchers explore young women's reflections on having a serious illness.[1] One of their main findings is that the women feel "off time"—out of sync with what they were taught it means to be young, because their bodies started breaking down much earlier than they'd expected them to.

One thirty-three-year-old woman who experienced menopausal symptoms from breast cancer treatment put it this way: the things that happen to an older woman are happening to you at the wrong time. Another person couldn't relate to the women she met with the same disease because they were all older and already had kids, even grandkids. They didn't know what it was like to be the only one struck by serious illness among young, carefree, illness-free friends.

And serious illness, the researchers explain, leads some women to renegotiate their expectations for their young-adult years and beyond. I've met women who, when they suddenly discover they have a disease, begin to distrust their immune systems, to feel betrayed by their own bodies, to worry about how they'll have to adapt—and to brace themselves for something else to "go wrong."

While plenty of people with a disability or health condition don't consider it something wrong at all and would find that term—*something wrong*—quite problematic, even offensive, it's one of the reactions I've encountered, both in myself and in others. When you're at a party one day and in the hospital the next, or were born with sickle cell anemia and later learn you have a tumor, it can make you wonder: What'll strike next?

There are many people who don't have this negative view of their bodies. I don't want to feed into a problematic narrative that everyone with a health issue is upset about it, as that would erase many people's lived experience.[2] At the same time, I can't pretend that I'm not upset about my surgeries or my cancer. I used to go on long runs every day and once found running the only way I could sort out my thoughts. I also used to have a thyroid. Back then, I could stay alive without relying on medicine. I can't pretend that I don't feel angry at the universe now that I can't do those things.

And for many young women, factoring in the ways they must adapt can be exhausting. The visits to doctors that no one else their age has to deal with. The way joint pain or surgery or a neurological change affects their relationship and career goals, their fears of being accepted or employed in a world run mostly by nondisabled people. For instance, as one study found, young people with lupus felt that their identity was now marred. The participants felt self-conscious and isolated. They believed that their bodies misrepresented them and that their ability to travel or find meaningful careers was more limited. "Well if I want to live overseas or something, or do backpacking," one twenty-six-year-old woman said, "I can't do it because if I run out of medication that's it, it's the end of the world for me."[3]

Feeling hemmed in by the way you need to adapt when all you want to do is go out and be young and explore can affect not just you, but how you interact with other people. And this is largely due to the biased way we are taught to view various bodies—and our lack of willingness, on a societal level, to accommodate them. If, say, a young woman always needs to be within an hour of a hospital, can she date someone who wants to visit remote spots in the wilderness? Can she explain why, although she loves camping, she no longer feels safe being out in the middle of nowhere, away from emergency care? Will the twenty-five-year-old she's on a date with understand if the woman needs to limit the number of blocks she walks because she has early-onset arthritis? Will anyone her age still think she's fun and lively if she tells a good story, then has to go lie down?

Of course, one day, everyone's bodies will decline. But if you're young—say, between eighteen and thirty-five—you don't expect it to happen yet. You are, as one young-adult cancer survivor puts it, suddenly facing "the tasks of youth with a challenged world view and a compromised physiology."[4] You're a woman who's barely out of high school or college, or you're thirty and supposedly at your sexual peak. You're in pain, or you need to be cut open, or your immune system is weak, or it's overly strong, or there's a tumor or a faulty valve, or your blood pressure is out of whack. You are strange to your "healthy" friends, who perhaps want to understand, but can't. You are strange to the older women you meet—women who cluck and say, "Too young."

And on top of that, what you keep hearing, whether you're single or partnered, is that you're already in danger of being ditched.

At Thanksgiving a few years ago, I told a cousin about my health issues, how they'd knocked me off course the past year. She was around fifty at the time and said I reminded her of herself in her twenties. Back then, she'd been an actress, a jazz singer, a young woman with a boyfriend. All that (with incredible cheekbones, I should add) when she was diagnosed with an autoimmune disease. At which point, she told me, her boyfriend chose to leave her.

My cousin's story was just one of many that sparked a feeling— the constant, dull fear of being left when illness creeps in. A fear that hummed in me when I went on dates, careful not to mention the surgery I'd undergo the following week. A fear that prevents many young women from even trying to meet someone, because who, after all, would want to kiss a body in early decay?

Fear isn't always based in reality. You can hold a spider that has no venom and realize how fragile it is. You can wade into a pool and see that, no, though the water laps past you toward the drain, you aren't sucked in with it.

But instead of proving that your worries are unsubstantiated, reality sometimes shows you just how warranted they might be.

Take Newt Gingrich. The story of how the politician ditched his wife when she was undergoing cancer treatment has stuck with me, and stuck with many of us. It's appeared in numerous newspapers, magazines, online stories, and broadcasts: Gingrich at the hospital with his daughters to see his then-separated wife, Jackie, right after her third cancer-related surgery. Gingrich demanding they move on with the divorce, even as Jackie lies in a hospital bed.[5]

And then, there's another one. Gingrich's second wife, Marianne, told ABC News that she, too, had been hit with a serious health issue just before her husband moved for divorce.[6] He had been in the room with her, she said, when the doctor diagnosed her with MS. Gingrich left her within a matter of months.

There's also Padma Lakshmi, the writer and *Top Chef* host who revealed that during her marriage to famed author Salman Rushdie, he had called her "a bad investment" because she had endometriosis.[7]

But it's not just about public figures. These stories come from everyday people, too.

A former colleague recently told me over tacos about a friend of hers from college, a young woman named Helena who had ovarian cancer in her twenties. Helena and her boyfriend were more or less engaged and very committed to each other. Deeply so. But after the ovarian cancer, her boyfriend broke off the relationship. The illness, he said—even though it was in remission—made him afraid of losing her. So he lost her on purpose instead.

As we finished our meal, I silently, reluctantly, added this last tale to my mental file. "That's exactly what I'm talking about," I said. "That's exactly what makes young women like me feel rejected, preemptively."

My old coworker wasn't done. There was a second half to the story, she said. Helena eventually dated someone new. Since they were falling for each other quickly, she decided to be up-front about her health. She told the guy that although she'd been in remission for a while and was healthy and cancer-free, there was still a small chance that she might not be able to have kids. Helena wasn't even sure about this possibility—for all she knew, she'd be just fine getting pregnant and delivering. But she wanted to let him know, just in case.

That guy broke up with Helena, too. He said he was falling for her hard, but couldn't commit to a woman who might not be able to give birth. So he left her. Two in a row.

A while later, I looked at the research. In 2001, researchers at the annual meeting of the American Society of Clinical Oncology reported on their study of heterosexual married couples where either the husband or the wife had a brain tumor. They said that men were almost ten times more likely to leave women with brain tumors than women were likely to leave men with the same disease.[8] Ten.

One of the researchers points out a staggering gender disparity with other illnesses, too, including MS and lung cancer. In the case of lung cancer, their research suggests that women are 5.7 times more at risk of divorce than men with the same diagnosis: "The risk factor [for divorce] is still high," the researcher says, "and it's still the men who walk away."[9]

The men who walk away.

I wanted to find more studies, ones that reflected more kinds of relationships—between people who aren't defined by marriage, and between partners of various genders and sexualities. At the same time, I knew that the existence of any studies on women and illness and relationships was a big deal. Research still skews toward the bodies and experiences of straight cisgender white men (for more on this problem, see part 4).

In another study, this one from 2015, researchers at Iowa State University looked at illness and divorce—inspired, they said, by Gingrich himself.[10] They wanted to see how cancer, heart disease, lung disease, and stroke affected heterosexual marriages. They found that in hetero couples, heart issues in a woman are associated with an elevated risk of divorce.[11] And the *New York Times*, in reporting on a 2009 study from the journal *Cancer*, put it this way: "Divorce Risk Higher When Wife Gets Sick." According to that study, conducted over several years by some of the same researchers who presented at the oncology conference, women who'd been diagnosed with a serious illness were nearly seven times more likely to become separated or divorced than similarly diagnosed men.[12]

I already knew this discrepancy existed, I thought. I knew this every time I went on a date with a guy, even if for me the ideal relationship wouldn't include marriage. I knew this from all the stories I'd heard; I knew it instinctively. The illness of one kind of partner—a woman—was treated differently than the illness of a man. And although having a medical issue strike at any age can be scary and painful, having it strike when your peers still think the word *young* means *immortal* makes things even more complicated. Researchers at the University of Utah, for instance, found that people with chronic illness in earlier adulthood, along with their spouses, may find the illness more stressful than do couples who are older.[13]

I'd harbored a vague hope for a while before admitting it to myself in words: that as I dated people and maybe found a partner of some sort, I would come across someone who had been through hard things, too. Maybe the person had had cancer or a joint condition. Yes, I was hoping that I would find someone whose body was "messed up" like mine. Or at least someone who, like me, had experienced the death of a young parent—anything that would make them understand what it's like to feel old and weary as a twentysomething.

My father's death might have made me weary even if it hadn't been connected to health. But when, after talking about suicide for years as his MS symptoms got worse, my father killed himself as a form of euthanasia, his death took everything out of me. I was mourning my dad and, I now realize, grappling with his attitudes toward disability. I respected his sense of autonomy over his own body when it was in extreme pain. I also now wonder, as I recall how ashamed he was at the ways he had to adapt to his disease, how much the cultural and legal history of telling people that their bodies are too shameful to live with affected his sense of self-worth. He used to say that "good" people didn't try to live through a debilitating disease—that only the "evil" ones cling to life. How much of that mind-set came from his growing up in a world where so-called ugly laws that banned people with disabilities on the street still existed—laws that weren't fully repealed until the 1970s?[14] How much did the wide sweep of eugenics, and a general attitude that society doesn't care about people with disabilities, play a role in how he viewed himself?

The complex nature of my dad's death aside, I knew that other young people might understand me a little more, even if their health was fine, if they'd gone through a similar family loss. I didn't want to wish something bad on a person. But if I met someone great who happened to also recognize their own mortality, unlike most of our young peers, I might not have to hide parts of myself. We'd feel, I thought, more like we were going through something together, not that one of us had to wait around while the other one dealt with her health shit. It'd be like a longer-term version of when you and someone you're

dating both get food poisoning. In fact, I thought, that kind of cama-
raderie didn't sound so bad. Not because feeling your stomach lining
turn to daggers is particularly fun, or because the complete disruption of your body is itself a fond memory. But when you and another
person are both sick with the same thing, at the same time, in the
same way, you bond. You enter a realm of sticky-clothes romance,
full of acrid sweat that might otherwise seem gross but in this moment
means you're together. There's the way you take turns doubling over,
listing out loud to each other which food might be the culprit. *Could
it have been the lo mein?* you ask. *Maybe. But we also had that ice
cream*, the other says. *I've never heard of food poisoning from mint
chocolate chip*—and so on, until one of you grabs your midsection in
pain. You share the same pain and the same bodily revolt. Both of you
are equally wretched, neither of you the killjoy.

In my junior year of college, my then boyfriend and I took a trip
to Costa Rica. Our relationship was somewhat nice, somewhat terrible. But we were in love, and so we found a tiny spice farm with a
few boarder rooms and took a three-hour bus ride on the side of a
cliff to get to the rural hostel. We helped plant watermelons, chopped
down sugarcane, and drove to a nature preserve to spot monkeys and
bright-colored crabs.

The vegetables in the sandwiches we ate one day must have been
washed with tap water, though: we woke up at four in the morning
clutching our middles and writhing in pain. For the next two days,
we expelled our meal into a toilet so rustic it had no door, though
it was attached to our room. Nothing could be less sexy. And yet,
this was the moment that our two-and-a-half-year partnership was
the strongest. It's what we reminisced about years later as the most
counterintuitively wonderful time in our coupledom. Shared physical
vulnerability, we learned, can become a bizarre aphrodisiac, a bond
that is gross and uncomfortable but ultimately positive.

Not so when it is just one of you and the health issue isn't
temporary.

"I'm not going to tell him *where* I'm sick," a student of mine said. We
were meeting to discuss a draft of hers after our evening journalism

class. And we were talking about how her recent absences were affecting not just her ability to keep up with classwork but also her personal life. Mara had undergone three surgeries in just one week. And she was trying to feel as normal as possible and do all her work despite her medical meltdown.

First, she said, she had felt a sudden terrible pain. A doctor performed a small procedure to remove a ruptured cyst. She didn't tell me where exactly the cyst was, but only said that it was somewhere too embarrassing to tell a guy.

Mara was nineteen, a sophomore, and focused on school and friends, even though her body often did strange, painful things that needed a rush of medical attention. So when she got back to school after the surgery, she tried to hang out with her classmates as if nothing had happened. But when the pain set in a few days later, she raced back to the doctor. The site had become infected, he said. He had to open her back up. When that procedure didn't quite work, either, the doctor told her to go to the hospital. He'd need to do a more complicated operation with general anesthesia.

Mara wasn't happy about the pain or about waking to oxygen tubes up her nose. But she is used to it now, she told me. Used to having a young woman's body that looks "normal" on the outside but has a whole lot of weird things within. She has severe irritable bowel syndrome, she said—but would never tell the boy she's been seeing: too gross. Who wants to hear about an irritable bowel, she thought, even if for her it means serious health consequences? She has to eat only known ingredients, can't have anything from the dining hall where her friends eat every night, and sometimes has a sudden bout for which she needs an emergency infusion of medicine.

Her father had offered to drive her around during the week of endless surgery on the part of her body she wouldn't mention. In case it hurts to sit, he'd said.

"Ewww," Mara said, as we stood in our classroom. "I don't want to talk to my dad about that!"

And she certainly didn't want to talk about it with the boy she'd been hooking up with, even though he kept asking her what was wrong.

"I lie all the time," Mara confided, after I told her that I've been through a hellish combination of illnesses at a young age, too. "Like when he asked me where I had surgery. I told him it was my upper leg. He doesn't need to know where it really is."

When young women with serious illness talk to each other privately, we tend to trade details of what we consider our grossest moments. *I had this tube up my nose and the anesthesiologist came in and I realized he was cute and my age!* Or, *I didn't want to explain to the guy on our fourth date that I had a giant strip of gauze absorbing pus from my stomach—so gross, right? So when we started to make out, I just said I was tired. Easier than having him see that.*

After participating in enough of these conversations, I've noticed how many of them center on sex and romance, or the glimmer of it. Will someone think I'm gross, and is that person already scrutinizing my body? As if women don't have enough to worry about.

I've also noticed that these conversations about grossing the other person out with one's health issues tend to be about men. What will this *guy* think when he sees/hears/feels my tube/history/scar? As someone who dated men for many years before realizing, a bit late in the game, that I'm far more gay than straight, I've noticed, anecdotally, some differences with dating women (or dating people who identify as nonbinary). While the fear of being rejected for my health issues has certainly not gone away completely, it was far more palpable with men. During the years that I went on dates exclusively with guys and thought that men were the only ones who could make me feel electric, I knew that I was expected to be *the woman* in the relationship. Even if these were the types of guys my friends and I considered feminist, or enlightened—men who don't consciously expect the woman to be a certain way—those deep cultural forces and beauty standards and gender roles were still there in the relationship, pinning us down.

That said, expectations for gender roles and bodies don't vanish just because neither of the people in a relationship is a man. Plenty of women who date other women or who date people who are nonbinary or genderqueer still feel self-conscious that their bodies may not work or look the way they think their partners would like. Or, they worry that they might be bothering their partners with their health issues. But there seems to be more of a precedent for cisgender men rejecting women for their health.

So when at twenty-six I undressed at Mount Sinai Hospital and got ready to have my thyroid cut out, being boyfriendless didn't seem so bad. A doctor was about to slice into my neck and pull out a cluster of small tumors and one of the organs that kept me alive. What a relief, in a way, not to have to explain it to a guy.

My anesthesiologist, it turned out, was in fact young and good-looking. And beyond that, he worked with patients and surgeries every day, which meant he understood, perhaps, that a person is not the most freakish of freaks just because she is young and in the hospital. As he stood in his blue mask above my bed in the presurgery room, I was suddenly embarrassed at how drawn my face must have looked after the required fast and how tired and scared I must have seemed. But I was also excited to meet an attractive person who maybe knew how to see past my health status.

"You're so small," the anesthesiologist said softly, as he and the rest of the medical team transferred me to the operating table. And somehow, in some misogynistically socialized part of my brain, *small* was a compliment, the moment was now happier, and the frightening procedure that could rob me of my vocal chords, if not fail to remove all the cancer, was now that much less scary.

A week went by. I thought a lot about how strange it was to live without a major organ, to rely on medicine that comes in a disposable plastic bottle, and to walk around with an empty neck.

The anesthesiologist called to see how I was doing post-procedure. Routine, perhaps. Then I remembered a conversation we'd had at the hospital. "So how exactly does anesthesia work?" I'd asked. "We're not completely sure," he'd replied.

As a writer, the question intrigued me—as did the anesthesiologist himself. I decided to challenge my idea of what women's bodies had to look like to be desirable. That, or I wanted some validation from a person who wasn't afraid of medical problems. So, after finding his e-mail address in the hospital directory, I sent him a message. I wanted to hear more about how doctors like him didn't understand the chemicals they used, I said. For a story I'd pitch to my editor.

In fact, I did want to write an article about anesthesiologists admitting that they don't quite know how things work, that the medicine they pump into you before surgery brings you into a state of unconsciousness in a somewhat mysterious way. But really, I had the idea that getting coffee to interview him would then turn into a date.

So I wrote what I hoped was a charming e-mail, admitting that the whole thing was a bit unorthodox. Here's where I work as a journalist, I said. Here's the kind of story I'd like to interview you for. And then, toward the end:

> In sum: I'd love to pick your brain (unfortunate pun) on both the science and the art of being a budding anesthesiologist. It does feel sliiiightly embarrassing to email someone who's (a) put a tube down my throat, (b) seen me in unflattering hospital garb, and (c) watched someone slice my neck. But hey, it can only go up from here, right?

The anesthesiologist agreed after checking with his supervisor. We met for coffee at a boring Starbucks he'd suggested. He wasn't, I realized, as cute without the blue face mask below his eyes, and he wasn't as cute, either, when I was in a less vulnerable position.

Slightly less vulnerable, that is. I was still his patient of a week ago and had a bright red slash across my neck where another doctor had scalpeled me. But this time I was upright, wearing more than paper, and not about to fall unconscious.

We had an okay discussion about anesthesiology—the science was more fascinating than he was, I decided—and ended up getting into some clichéd philosophical talk about the physical substrate of the mind. He kind of went on and on. It wasn't so interesting.

When he suddenly checked the time and had to go, I got the feeling he had a girlfriend waiting for him to make dinner. But I was far from crestfallen. Although I'd have bragging rights as the only one of my friends who'd ever asked out a person from her surgical team, this real-life version of the man seemed far from the one who'd felt sparkling in the weird, sterile hospital room.

"I asked out my anesthesiologist!" I announced to several friends. It felt easier than telling my fellow twentysomethings what was really going on: *I am exhausted. My scar stings the walls of my throat when I talk. I'm scared of the next phase of treatment.*

It felt more relevant to say I had tried to squeeze romance out of a funny-sad circumstance.

A few days later, I was back at work and mentioned the mysteries-of-anesthesia story to one of the senior editors. I told her how I'd interviewed my own doctor, who had admitted that even he didn't know how anesthetics or unconscious states worked. How bizarre, I said, that specialists all over the world control our brains during operations, leading us somewhere between sleep and death, without really understanding how.

Not enough of the magazine's readers could relate to having surgery and anesthesia, the editor said. The topic just isn't relevant to a wider audience.

Somewhere in me, I knew she was wrong. I could have told her that in the United States, we collectively have fifty-one million inpatient surgeries a year. That many people—all kinds of people, including many of our readers—have operations. But I let it go, because in that moment, I believed her: that somehow I was an outlier and that health wasn't a mainstream issue.

A month later, my scar was still bright red, raw. *Oh god, what's that slash across your neck!?* a few people asked. It seemed to alarm everyone who spotted it. I didn't want to go to a dinner or another gathering with strangers, even though I finally had the energy for it. I didn't want to have to answer the question.

But there was a reading I wanted to attend at the Housing Works bookstore in SoHo, and I decided it was worth being out with my red-slashed neck. I went with a work friend and felt momentarily like a young woman who hadn't just undergone cancer surgery.

After the reading, there was a casual after-party. The booksellers shuffled us toward a nearby bar, and that's where I met Simon. That's where I hoped that the bar was too dim for him to see my scar.

A few wonderful dates later, I was vibrating with liking Simon more than I'd liked anyone in years—Simon, who knew nothing of

how difficult my twenties had been thus far, with my throat closing up unexpectedly, several near-death moments, and now cancer. I
couldn't fathom telling him about the radioactive hazard I would become in just two weeks or the strict diet I'd have to follow every day
leading up to the treatment.

"Just fib and tell him you'll be out of town for a while," my friend
Janice suggested. She, like me, seemed vivacious on the outside while
internally she was gnarled with medical problems. She'd had heart
surgery three times, starting in college, but you wouldn't know it
talking to her. Not without glimpsing the armory of heart pills she
kept at home or the part of her chest that she covered with clothes.
And like me, Janice dreaded the smashing of her healthy-looking facade. She had gone on a date a few days before her last surgery and
laughed and distracted herself and told the guy nothing. It seemed
natural to her that if Simon and I had spent just a few days together,
I didn't need to tell him my whole story.

The problem was, I reminded Janice, I have never been good at
lying. Even when I want to, I fail. I leak truth.

"Remember that awful date with the illustrator?" I asked. Oof—
Janice remembered. A few years earlier, in a foreshadowing of my
dilemma with Simon, I'd met a guy in the middle of a strange, scary
medical period. He was a cute illustrator. When he asked me out to
dinner, I couldn't fathom telling him that I was recovering from being
a few seconds from death when my throat had closed up out of nowhere. Because really, how could I reveal that I'd come within thirty
seconds of dying, been revived at the emergency room, and now was
allowed to eat white rice, plainly cooked eggs, spinach, and one species of apple until doctors figured out if there was a food trigger?

So I scoured the menus of restaurants near my office and found a
crappy place that offered eggs for dinner. This restaurant pretended
to be nice but was really a glorified diner, just without the interesting
kitsch. All it had was bad food and a touristy atmosphere. Embarrassing. But it had eggs, and so I wouldn't risk dying, and that, well,
seemed key. I lied and told the illustrator I'd heard great things about
the eatery. Then, when we got there, I feigned surprise that the place
was a dump—I swore that someone had recommended it. "Let's just

try it, I guess?" was how I weakly put it, even though the illustrator and I were within feet of better restaurants.

I watched him frown at his plate of mediocre food. Then I spent the whole dinner wondering if the cooking oil coating my spinach omelet was safe for me to eat. My doctors might think even this was too risky, I realized. And if a hidden ingredient did in fact trigger something dangerous, I'd have to tell my date, after all, what my deal was, and he would need to stab my thigh with an epinephrine injector to save my life.

The date didn't go very well.[15]

So, back to the crisis at hand, I said to Janice. Her idea to tell Simon that I was on vacation instead of in cancer treatment might work for somebody else, but I wasn't that somebody. With the illustrator, I hadn't even been able to get through one meal based on lies. And if Simon and I went on a few more dates, we'd reach the day that my radioactive treatment preparation would start, when I would have to cook all my food, even snacks, and couldn't have many basic ingredients. On that day, at the very latest, I'd have to explain things to him, instead of trying to cover them up.

It was a Monday night. Simon and I met after work. Both of us surged with new infatuation, but only I surged with the anxiety of an unhappy secret. Simon had just learned about the historic landmarks in his neighborhood by taking a city-sponsored tour. Tonight, he took me on his version of it, pointing to the same hidden gargoyles and paint-flecked arches that the professional tour guides had. His ability to describe architecture from the late nineteenth century without the cockiness I too often found in potential mates had me swooning. Here was the rare young man who had a host of bright tail feathers yet didn't seem to notice them, let alone preen.

I didn't want to spoil the ease of the evening with my news. But I had to, or else I'd truly have to pretend to be away for weeks and weeks and describe a vacation to cover up a hospital stay. So when we got back to Simon's living room, I clenched my shoulders and suggested that he sit down. My underarms were noxious with anxiety sweat. I didn't care about the sweat, though, as long as I could say what I needed to and hopefully not be another woman with a story of being ditched.

"The scar is from thyroid cancer," I said. "My surgery was just a few weeks ago. And while that answers your question about why my neck looks so red, there's actually more."

This was the year that the Fukushima nuclear reactor had erupted in Japan. Simon and I had both seen the footage on every news channel: the haunting images of a damaged reactor, the people scurrying away from danger. Reporters described how crowds of Japanese citizens rushed to take iodine pills, a method to block their thyroids from absorbing radioactivity from the disaster. Weirdly, I told Simon, the way you treat thyroid cancer is by doing the opposite. You swallow a radioactive form of iodine that doesn't block radioactivity, but causes it.

In just a few weeks, I explained, I'd take the opposite of the pill that people near Fukushima were taking. A team of doctors would make me radioactive on purpose in the hopes of killing off any cancerous thyroid cells left over after surgery. It was bizarre enough without Fukushima, but the timing made it much stranger.

After explaining all of this, I paused. Simon was quiet. I took this to mean he was taken aback. How could a thirty-year-old guy want to be part of this? How could anyone following the news want to sleep with a twenty-six-year-old woman who was not running from but imbibing radioactivity?

"Thank you for telling me," he said. It was a whisper.

"But aren't you freaked out?" I asked. "I'm going to be radioactive!"

"I'm fascinated more than freaked out," he said. "And anyhow, 'Radioactive Michele' sounds like a superhero name." He smiled.

So I told him there was still more. For the fourteen days leading up to my mutant state, I couldn't eat food prepared by anyone else lest it contain a trace of iodine. The doctor of nuclear medicine—there was such a thing, I informed Simon, and the sci-fi nature of the phrase *doctor of nuclear medicine* had shocked me, too—said I could not even think of going to restaurants. I could not even eat plain rice from a takeout place because it surely contained iodized salt. And when I cooked for myself, which was the only option next to eating raw fruit all day, I couldn't use egg yolks or milk or cheese or butter or pasta sauce or a host of other things that might have comforted me. None of that, no comfort.

And, so, no dinner dates. If I had even a dusting of food with naturally occurring iodine, it would jeopardize my thyroid cells' ability to absorb the radioactive form of the element in a few weeks. I could not even go for a cocktail, the doctor said, in case some salt crept into the glass. I could not make a mistake.

I'd also have to go off the medicine that replaced my thyroid hormones for several weeks. That would make my body and mind slow down. I wouldn't be able to walk outside much or concentrate—maybe not even read.

Simon, again, seemed unfazed. I was the one who could barely make eye contact, who was sweating, and who assumed that by the time I sat in my hospital isolation room, Simon would be out to dinner with some other young woman, one who couldn't be nicknamed Mothra. But he was fine with everything, he said. He only felt bad that I had to go through it—and that I was even worried he'd run away.

There's a reason for that, I told Simon. There's a reason I thought you might flee.

———

During my research, I meet a woman named Vita, who identifies as a straight, half-Mexican woman of color. Vita was twenty-three when she was diagnosed with multiple sclerosis. After flings and more casual hookup partners, she tried dating. She had read blog posts about people hiding their disability, but that wasn't her style.

There was a guy she'd worked with occasionally, someone she'd known for a number of years and had always thought was cute. They went on a first date and then a second. In the spirit of not hiding things, she mentioned her MS.

Vita and her longtime crush started to make out. And then, in the middle of making out, he pushed her away.

"I can't do this. It's too intense," he said.

"What's too intense?" Vita asked.

"What you shared with me earlier," he told her. And he left.

Vita brings me back to that moment. She felt unworthy then and for a long while after. And she remembers thinking, "Are people going to leave me over this shit?"

———

Vita is far from the only one whose illness has ended a relationship. When I was three, my family moved to a new neighborhood in Manhattan. My parents and, eventually, I would occasionally chat with a pair of women who lived nearby. They said they were sisters, though they had different last names and different faces. We were neighborly enough that the two women would deposit small wondrous gifts in a bag on our doorknob each time a holiday came around. I would get chocolate bunnies on Easter and chocolate coins on Chanukah and, once—especially decadent—a jewelry-making kit replete with real stone beads for my birthday. They were Angie and Margaret, or Angie-and-Margaret, a unit of some sort. At some point, I realized that Angie and Margaret probably weren't sisters or even half-sisters or stepsisters. But I didn't press it.

Once, when I was already out of college and visiting my mother, I ran into Margaret. I mentioned some of the severe health issues I was dealing with. And then Margaret, realizing I understood what it was like to beat back health issues and go to doctor after doctor, reciprocated with her own illness, a tricky beast that caused rashes on her face and exhaustion from the sun and a general lack of ability to digest foods. She'd been dealing with these health complications since she was in her twenties.

Then Margaret mentioned that her health had caused a breakup, ruined a major relationship when she was younger. She mentioned it in passing, but the breakup was clearly momentous. She spoke as if she wanted me to ask more about it.

So finally, a few years later, I ask. I invite Margaret out for tea so we can talk about her health issues and so she can explain how they'd foiled many of her plans for the past thirty-five years. But because she's photosensitive and constantly exhausted, Margaret invites me over for some at-home tea instead. While she ushers me to an overstuffed chair in the duo's pastel living room, Angie—the woman she has been living with for all these decades—retreats to the bedroom to give us privacy. "But," Margaret says wryly, "there's nothing that Angie doesn't already know."

I've come over to ask this neighbor-turned-friend how an illness in her early twenties had changed who she was. But before I can ask anything, Margaret starts to explain. No, she and Angie aren't sisters, she says. When they first moved here in the 1970s, they told everyone in the building that they were, because Angie was afraid that people would talk if they said otherwise.

But no, they aren't a couple, either. They're both *heterosexual*— Margaret enunciates the word—and they met at church. It's irritating and frustrating, Margaret tells me, that people assume they're gay.

I wouldn't have cared either way, I want to tell her, but I can see that to Margaret the distinction is important. They've been living together all these years, she said, because they're both "spinsters"— her word.

They've been living together because her illness changed everything.

In 1976, Margaret tells me, she was dating a man named Tim. They were the kind of couple who were giddy and in love and wanted to keep growing together. She was a nurse and twenty-six; he was a third-year law student and twenty-five. They had both, as she puts it, "kissed enough frogs to know that we were hysterically happy together." So they decided to get married. And to celebrate their engagement, they planned a special night out.

That Friday evening, as Margaret waited for Tim to pick her up so they could go toast to their future, she got a call from a doctor following up from a medical test. He said they'd found a tumor in her bladder. She would have to be admitted that weekend for surgery.

Then, Tim arrived.

Margaret was standing there in her little black dress, and Tim had on a tuxedo. They planned to celebrate with a concert at Carnegie Hall and then a meal at the Russian Tea Room.

Margaret was shaken. Her grandmother had died of bladder cancer, and maybe she, Margaret, was next. But she and Tim still went to the concert. Two days later, she went to the hospital and had the tumor removed. Luckily, it was only pre-malignant. She'd have to follow up with testing every three months and would need a cystoscope—a tube that snakes through your urethra and up to your bladder to take biopsies—but for now, she was fine.

She was relieved that she didn't have full-blown cancer, even if she'd still have to go through uncomfortable biopsies every three months. She and Tim had already started planning their wedding— as had Tim's mother, a wealthy woman who loved the idea that Margaret, a fellow Irish Catholic, might steer her son back to the church. Margaret was peppy and book-smart and clean scrubbed, she says, and Tim's mother couldn't wait for the two to marry and have kids.

But when Tim's mother found out about the pre-malignant tumor and the testing every three months, it was as if a switch had flipped. The mother assumed, without having any medical knowledge, that Margaret wouldn't be able to give birth. And as much as she had loved Margaret as a soon-to-be daughter-in-law, she suddenly turned on her.

"She's sick," Tim's mother told her son. "She's not going to be able to have kids." And like that, she threatened the couple. She told them that if they chose to stay together, she would cut them off. All because Margaret would need some follow-up screenings.

At this point in Margaret's story, I am locking my diaphragm, holding my breath, as she recounts what happened. I know what's going to come next. But hearing how little things have changed since the 1970s, I tighten my body. I armor it.

Things got worse, Margaret tells me. Tim's mother wanted Margaret, this young woman she had already welcomed into the family, to go away now that she had health problems. But Tim loved Margaret and wanted to spend his life with her. He fought against his mother's wishes. And so his mother, sensing that she couldn't force her son to leave the love of his life, tried to leverage her wealth to give the couple an ultimatum: Margaret could marry Tim, against the family's wishes, but if so, they must try to have children right away. If Margaret wasn't successfully pregnant within a year, she and Tim would have to separate.

And for her time, Margaret would get half a million dollars, as a "consolation." Meaning, she had a year to prove herself worthy of the family by producing a child. Otherwise, she'd be paid to leave.

"They saw a baby maker," Margaret says. Tim's family had welcomed her—even rushed to include her in their son's life and talked about wedding venues—and now they were trying, soap-opera style, to pay her off. And all because she needed medical tests.

As I'm listening, my eyes fill up. I think about Simon's parents finding out about all of my medical problems and what their reaction might be. As Margaret coolly recounts the rest of her story, I blink and keep listening and pretend to be okay.

Tim fought back, Margaret says. He thought his mother's offer of money to force a separation was preposterous. But although he wanted to stay with Margaret, he eventually crumpled. His parents did not back down, and he started to realize that they really would cut him off if he didn't do as they wished. He began to see a therapist. He wasn't himself.

Margaret could see that as much as Tim loved her, their united front of Margaret-and-Tim was slipping. She realized that his parents would win. Margaret's would-be mother-in-law had rejected her and offered an absurd amount of money, and there was no taking the deed back. So Margaret told Tim it just wasn't going to work out. And two months before their wedding date, the relationship was over.

I've known Margaret for several decades at this point, but I still can't let her story end the way I know it will. I know she lives with Angie; I know there is no Tim in her life. But I find myself fighting back against the narrative.

Didn't his parents see that you and Tim loved each other? I ask. What kind of person plans a wedding for her son and then tries to pay the bride to walk away?

I am a staunch advocate of living however one wants to live: without a partner, with a partner, with more than one partner, with any gender or sexual identity. Anything. But I cringe when Margaret calls herself a spinster. I want to believe she is happy living the way it worked out, with her and Angie sharing a platonic bedroom, two small beds, this living room with the blankets they've crocheted, occasional squabbling. But I can see that she is back in the 1970s as she talks and she is back in that black dress and she is hurt.

Margaret is a calm, logical type. She describes herself as thinking over feeling and says she is fine with how things turned out. But she had loved Tim and wanted to be with him for the rest of her life.

And after she felt forced to end the relationship to avoid the situation with his family, she was still tied to the regular cancer screenings that had scared off Tim's mother. She began to fear having to tell another man about her health. She told the next man she met nothing of her medical history.

Five years later, another illness struck. This time it was the autoimmune disease that still gives Margaret digestive and connective-tissue problems. When the disease worsened, she tells me, she withdrew from her sexual life. She says it matter-of-factly, just like that, but there's emotion beneath the even tone.

It's about feeling like you don't quite make the mark anymore, Margaret says. "And it's not like you're looking in the mirror at your boobs or worrying about an extra ten pounds or anything. This is a really heavy load, and you have to be able to cope with the scrutiny and the stigma and all the uncertainty that it brings." And, she adds, "it never leaves."

It never does leave. Some women I know have been healthy now for many years following surgery, but still feel that a glimpse of the scar is enough to scare away potential mates. And in my case, even after I revealed to Simon my cancer, the surgery, and the strange, frightening radioactive quarantine, I wasn't at all done. One day, he finally saw my bag lying open, the bright yellow EpiPens sticking out. And another day, while we were out hiking, my hip pain became so extreme that I had to stop and explain why.

Each time I opened up about another health problem that a woman my age isn't expected to have, I wondered if it would be the last health problem Simon would be able to absorb. Maybe, after hearing enough of the truth about my health, he'd leave and find a young woman without such a jangled body and its threat of shutting down any minute.

"Why would the mast-cell thing that makes your throat close up freak me out?" he would say, and I would laugh, because I couldn't figure out why it didn't.

Even if you don't have an illness that could erupt anytime and kill you in a matter of seconds—a quick and chilling condition like my

tendency toward anaphylactic shock—feeling like a medical specimen is decidedly unsexy, somehow the opposite of whatever we're
taught is womanhood. Writer Lisa Glatt gives an image of this in
a prose poem. The poem's speaker is being examined by a male gynecologist after her mother has died of breast cancer. "I'm thinking
that it's a wonderful thing my love and I don't have sex on a table
like this," Glatt writes, "that he doesn't see me in this light, that he
doesn't peer in with sticks and tools."[16]

On my end, Simon always said he'd be happy to come with me to
the doctor if I needed him, that he didn't mind seeing me on a table
like this, in this light, peered into with sticks and tools. But whenever
I've taken him up on it, I've had a flash of regret. I'd lie down on the
examining table and think, as I lowered my head, that Simon looked
so upright, so invulnerable, sitting in a chair, looking on. I know,
logically, that he is just as vulnerable as I am, that all of us are, at
various times, because we're bodies, and we're aging. But it seemed
incredible to me that he loved me enough to deal with all my medical
appointments, still loved the strange specimen I became as the doctor
leaned over me in the dark, an ultrasound machine flickering images
of my post-tumor throat, my neck slathered in conductive goo. Like
Glatt and many people with health issues, these types of moments
feel vulnerable, unappealing—even "unladylike," an idea I've been
trying my whole conscious life to dismantle but that nonetheless sti-
fles young women everywhere.

Though I had already told Simon about my most ominous health
conditions, there were some additional minor ones I just didn't feel
like explaining. But one day, a year and half into our relationship,
we were about to order delivery for dinner. Knowing that this was
yet another reveal, I said that I needed to eat something neutralizing
because of my "old-man heartburn." I explained that it was a condition I had developed after going to school near the World Trade Center attacks. A federal health study had found the condition in many
9/11 survivors, and yet somehow it still seemed like an old man's
disease—even though it came from something solemn and sad and
was unrelated to gender or age. Simon was caring and asked if I was
okay. I ascribed the slight look of awe in his eyes to his not believing
that this woman he was dating had Yet Another Medical Problem.

I was about to blurt out *Sorry*, then caught myself. Why was I sorry? Was it contagious? No. Was it ruining our night? No.

"It's funny," I told Simon. "I was about to say sorry about having heartburn, but then realized that didn't make sense."

"Yeah, that doesn't make sense," he said in a gentle tone. "Why would you apologize for your body hurting?"

He had a point. But it somehow went against everything we learn as women, as girls. I wanted to apologize for being a nuisance, for saddling him with so much medical crap. Instead, I told him that my heartburn had to do with a flap in my digestive tract not keeping the acids down.

The next day, I saw Simon again. "How's your flap?" he asked.

It struck me as so uncharacteristically wonderful that a person, a guy I was dating, would ask such an endearing and thoughtful question about my embarrassing condition, that I had to save it. I wrote it down.


In a *Bellevue Literary Review* essay that recalls the author's sense of self at age twenty as she tried to be an average college student one year after receiving a lifesaving heart transplant, Adina Talve-Goodman opens with a hookup.[17] She and the boy have whiskey, they kiss, and she asks him to spend the night. As they're undressing, he sees the scar down the middle of her chest and traces the keloids along the pink line. "What's this?" he asks. She remembers the conversation:

"I had a heart transplant," I said.
"When?"
"A year ago."
"Oh."
I waited for him to ask the usual questions: why did you need it, are you okay now, what about the donor.
"You have *great* boobs," he said.

After they hook up, Talve-Goodman examines all her surgical scars in the mirror and seems pleased—even a little grateful—to have slept with a guy, just as any other college student might do, despite the striking map on her torso. Whereas the boob comment could have seemed callous to someone else, in this scenario, with this health history, it was elating. She was still attractive despite all the scars, despite the scary sound of *heart transplant*. Still kind of "normal," young, fun.

The next morning, the boy tells her he'd be happy to help her practice lines that night before her play rehearsal. Then he heads to class.

"He was probably smoking a cigarette outside the library not knowing the gift he had given me by not asking questions," she writes, "and treating my body like I hadn't been split down the middle and pieced back together."

The line echoes what I've heard from nearly all the young women I've interviewed: a relief in finding a partner, long-term or for just one night, who doesn't focus on your illness. Who acknowledges your scars or your crutches or your other visible signs of health issues without letting it change the mood and without making you into a freak. Who, like this young man, compliments you, even if just superficially, and boosts your self-image.[18] Such a connection provides relief even if, like me, you wish that the way others talk about your sex appeal didn't influence how much you like yourself, or that your self-image had absolutely nothing to do with whether you find a mate—if, that is, you're looking for one. After all, there are many people who want to live on their own and don't want to be in a relationship: people whom social scientist Bella DePaulo calls "'single at heart'—those who live their best, most authentic and most meaningful lives by living on their own."[19] In her vital research on being single by choice and the discrimination heaped on those who choose not to date, DePaulo makes it clear that not everyone wants to have sex or find long-term romantic partners and that we tend to make false, harmful assumptions about people who live single lives.

That said, among the women I've interviewed, talk of health or disability often led quickly to talk of dating and sex. For young women who do want to pursue mates, body image and romantic life can get tangled. While many of us wish we got a hundred percent of our feelings of self-worth or attractiveness from within ourselves and were glowing with much-touted self-love, research shows that the way other people view and respond to women with chronic illness "has an important effect on their construction of self-identity."[20] We may want to feel fiercely self-empowered and not beholden to anyone else's expectations or opinions, but those expectations and opinions do affect us. Although, statistically speaking, young women make up a huge portion of some common diseases' demographics, we as a culture still find it strange and shocking or gross or weird when a young woman has a health condition.

"Not all men can deal with scars," a friend of mine said once. She is unusually stunning, this friend, smart and charming and someone whom men are always hopelessly drawn to, but even she has had the same experience. She undresses for the first time in front of a man and he sees a line down her chest from a long-ago surgery and he just can't.

"Doesn't that make sense, though, that you'd maybe not be as revved up to have sex if the person you're about to sleep with has a visible health condition?" a good friend asks. Having heard some of the stories I've gathered, he agrees that a lot of the men in these situations acted monstrously. And he himself has been on a few first dates with women who disclosed serious health issues. Endearingly, he'd come to me after each of the dates to ask, "Am I jerk because I'm maybe not so excited about a woman who's just had cancer or who's had surgery on a major organ?"

What he's getting at, he says, is that "some dudes are just awful." But, he points out, maybe there's some middle ground between acting like a total asshole—pushing someone away as you're kissing them—and having no qualms whatsoever about someone's body?

"That's a good question," I say. "Hmm. I don't think you're automatically an asshole just because you wonder about someone's health. I mean, I know that the women you've met who have medical stuff did make you think a little differently about whether or not to date them, and I've known you for years and I know you're not a jerk."

"I dunno, maybe I am!" he says. "But maybe there's some kind of evolutionary thing—like, you want a mate who's healthy. . . ."

"Yeah," I say, "there's definitely evolutionary psychology research around this stuff, but some of it's really interesting, and some of it sounds kind of sexist. Like some dudes decided that everyone is heterosexual and women have to look a certain way, and here is why we procreate—only with certain types of beauty emphasized more than others."

"Yeah, yikes," my friend says. "And then it can start to sound like eugenics."

"I think part of the problem," I say, "is that lots of people do seem to act in a shitty way once they find out about the other person's health history, and part of it is that there just don't seem to be as many *women* pushing *men* away because of their health. I'm sure some women have pushed guys away because the guys got sick, and I know there are guys who *don't* push women away. Nor am I some perfect human who doesn't notice someone's health. I'm sure I've had a visible reaction when I've gone to share a plate of mashed potatoes with someone and then noticed that they have a cold sore. But when it comes to ditching someone over health things, all signs point to this being an overwhelmingly male-dominated sport."

Indeed, it can suck to have chronic pain or an autoimmune disease you didn't ask for, or to try to navigate a subway system that isn't wheelchair-friendly when you're just trying to get to your friend's house—and it can suck regardless of your gender or age. But when young women are living with something medical, it's in direct opposition to what we're told we should be like: airbrushed beacons of sparkling youth. We seem young and vibrant looking, but on closer inspection, we're some kind of dud. We're attractive, but only up to a point. The oh-I-didn't-know-you-had-heart-surgery point. The point where sex partners, especially male sex partners, silently take in the history of our bodies and shift in their desire. Or, more deeply, in the way they even relate to us as people, as fellow young adults. Maybe we remind them that twentysomethings are not as invincible as we are led to believe.

Sometimes, the revulsion that young women dread is palpable: someone really does push us away mid-makeout because we have an autoimmune disease. But sometimes, even if the rejection isn't there, the prospect of it plays almost as large a role. In her essay about life as a twenty-year-old organ-transplant patient trying to have sex and experience college life, Talve-Goodman dismisses her own good experience with the guy she's hooked up with.

The guy had treated her body like any attractive woman's body, sure. "But now he knew that I walked around that campus with a perpetually broken chest plate and a very loud heart. And for that reason," she writes, "I didn't want to see him again."[21]

It's a common theme I've heard from young women: not wanting to expose your health vulnerability to someone you're already emotionally or sexually vulnerable with—even if that person seems on the surface to be fine with your scar or your illness or your explanation. Best not to have to explain in the first place, some of the young women I've met think. Best to avoid the reveal if you can, and keep projecting the idea of a fun, "normal" woman who's interesting but not a burden. Each time I had to reveal a health issue to Simon, I worried, even though he seemed unfazed.

April, who identifies as a white, queerish, cisgender woman in her late twenties, has had more than a dozen surgeries throughout her life, starting from a young age. Esophageal reconstructive surgery when she was born, a string of other operations when she was a kid, heart surgery when she was around twenty-one, and a pacemaker when she was twenty-four. We sit at the big kitchen table she shares with two roommates as she tries to count all the times a doctor has cut her open.

"My body is just covered in scars," she says. If she's with someone and doesn't have a shirt on, the scars are visible, no getting around it. When she's topless, she judges people: "I judge people if they ask me questions. I judge people if they don't ask me questions." Most of her experiences with sex partners have been positive, she tells me, but the reveal used to annoy her more. "I think now at least I feel comfortable in my body," she says, "like, I like my scars. Actually, I just got a tattoo along one of my scars."

The problem, though, is that even if she appreciates her skin these days, the marks from surgery reveal her health history, whether or not she's ready to reveal it. As she puts it, "It's on my body, and it's there for the world to see and question."

When it comes to spending the night with someone, scars aren't the only issue. Because of her esophageal condition, she needs to sleep on an incline. Otherwise, she's in pain. And even though it hurts for her to stay over on someone else's flat mattress, she does it. "I've been single for the past year, and so I've been dating," she says. "There's going to a bar and having a drink, and that usually can inflame my esophagus, and then let's say I decide to sleep with that person . . . dealing with the nighttime logistics can be pretty uncomfortable or painful." So she opts to act like a "regular" person on a date in her twenties, to hide her medical needs, to drink the drink that will hurt her, then sleep in the bed that will hurt her more, rather than explain to the person she's spending the night with. "It's like me sucking it up," she says.[22]

———

Days before I would go to the hospital for hip surgery and leave with holes in my thigh from where the scalpel had been, with no ability to walk without crutches for weeks, I was on a date. He was a musician named Mike, and we were talking and flirting and kissing and talking more, and he asked me if I would go out with him again a few days later. I paused. I couldn't, I knew, not because I wasn't interested in him, but because I would be laid up, immobile, probably in excruciating pain.

I had undergone this hip surgery before, in college. Not only was it awful, but it also sounded extremely unsexy. Having a problem with this part of your body made people say thoughtless, mildly hurtful things, like, "Wait, your hip?" or, "I thought only grandmas had hip surgery." Now this attractive guy wanted to make out in a few days, and I had to tell him yes except no, because I'd be having surgery.

Here again, I could have lied. I could have done what my journalism student does to avoid talking about gross-sounding body things with the guy she sleeps with. But I didn't. I chose not to, whether it was to prove that I was still a worthwhile person despite my health issues or because I am just bad at not telling the truth.

"Well, this is weird, but I'm actually having hip surgery on Monday," I said.

I expected that look of revulsion. I filled the silence like I always do when a person I've just met is learning something new or surprising about me. I made some awkward mumbly comment, like, "Kind of gross, I know, but it's not just for old ladies, haha," the *haha* coming out stilted and probably giving away that my throat was brink-of-crying tense.

Mike said only nice things. He didn't make some remark about grandmas. He just told me, as a way of commiserating or taking the weirdness out of the moment, that he had had mouth surgery once and, as he put it, "That's way grosser."

All that put me at ease. As did one comment I thought about for a while after: "You're having hip surgery, but I mean, you're still hot," which Mike delivered with a sheepish smile. Like the guy who compliments Adina Talve-Goodman on her great boobs, Mike meant it. Much as I wished I didn't need this kind of validation from a guy, it came across as a kind of warm, you-are-a-human-and-not-a-medical-oddity comment. Even though I normally got upset when men objectified women, in this moment, I felt relieved.

After a week of such staggering pain that I often stayed in one chair the whole day, I was ever so slightly better. I peeled off my day-old pajamas, covered the thick bandage on my hip with plastic so I could shower, and got dressed. I wanted to feel wanted. And in that moment, a deep-seated concept of what that entailed swam to the surface: curves. Although historically I have flitted between more androgynous outfits and the occasional tight vintage frock, there was no question tonight. I would wear a wiggly 1950s dress that was fitted at the waist—but just roomy enough at the hips that it showed my curves without pressing too hard against my bandage. The dress was like armor, protecting my bodily insecurities—a costume, as all clothing is. I wasn't sure if I was wearing the tight dress for me or for Mike, to show him that I was indeed still hot or to convince myself.

The subway was off-limits for another few weeks while I healed, so I maneuvered myself, with some pain, into a taxi and met Mike at a Thai place in Manhattan. Even with his comment about my hotness, I couldn't face, at twenty-five, the prospect of a new date seeing me on crutches. So I left them at home and promised myself, and my wary mother, that I would walk no more than from the curb to the restaurant.

Naturally, it didn't work out that way, and in the course of limping down several streets to go to a jazz club after dinner, I may have further damaged a major tendon, all in an attempt to show just how hot-and-not-gross I could be. And my limping earned me another compliment from my date. "You're walking pretty well for someone who just had surgery!" Mike said. He looked genuinely impressed. I said something self-deprecating and didn't tell him about the searing pain.

Mike was telling the truth about still being attracted to me. We decided to go to his place, and I slept over. But one hot date after my hip had been cut open couldn't undo or shield me from the way everyone else seemed to find it disturbing: this young woman robbed of her sprightliness and hobbling around because of her hip.

In the end, I got a long e-mail from Mike. He wrote that he was interested in me, but could tell I wasn't "the one" (a concept I didn't subscribe to but that he did).

I just wanted someone who made me feel like I was a young woman in the first place and not some monstrosity. I didn't need the person to think I was *the* one. So I replied to him. I just wanted to understand, I wrote: Was he attracted to me, or not, because after all his comments before my surgery and the way we'd hooked up afterward, I had thought he was saying he was.

I am attracted to you, he replied.

I was relieved. I didn't think we were serious-relationship material, either. I just needed to know that it wasn't about my hip.

In the elevator a few weeks later, a guy in his early thirties asked me why I was on crutches. His tone was bright, maybe even flirtatious.

He opened with, "Knee injury?"

"Oh, I had hip surgery a few weeks ago," I said. And then, remembering how people usually reacted to it, added brightly, with a smile, "It's not just for old ladies!"

The guy, who wore athletic clothes, was visibly repulsed. Disgust that he probably didn't mean to show flitted over his face.

"Oh." He scrunched his nose.

Then, in a withering tone: "You should just tell people it's your knee."


The way that man in the elevator scrunched his nose at me replays in my head every time I start to think that maybe we're all worrying about nothing. There are stories like Vita's and Helena's, Newt Gingrich's ex-wives' and my cousin's, where men started backing out because of health issues. But as much as those stories are the ultimate cause of my fear, it's the accumulation of smaller memories of disgust that stay with me. The elevator moment makes me mad, and sad, every time.

And from my teenage years, there's a TV image that crept into my mind and has had trouble finding its way out: a commercial for Bioré Deep Cleansing Pore Strips. Those little winged adhesive things you stick to your nose or your forehead that are supposed to pull out blackhead zits.

What I remember most is the look of disgust on the actress's face when she saw what had been living in her skin. She looked repulsed by her own body, then relieved at being that much "purer" after the facial treatment.

If I had endless time and a federal grant and a lab of social scientists, I know one of the studies I would do. I'd take a sample of television commercials related to personal care products and measure the looks of disgust on the actors' faces. Disgust is, after all, not just any facial expression, but one of only six (or, some say, four) that psychologists associate with a universal human emotion.[23] It can be measured and mapped: a certain wrinkle of the nose (like the man in the elevator), a certain movement of the lip, raised cheeks.[24] I'd find out how many ads in a random sample show a woman disgusted by her own body. Her nose zits or her razor bumps or her facial hairs or her frizzy hair or her split ends or, of course, her weight. Her crow's-feet. Her belly. Her butt.

I can't easily conduct such a study. Just to find all those television commercials and get a randomized sample would take time. But when we, as women, think back to the commercials we grew up with, it may not be random at all. What stands out? Did our brains store those revulsion-filled ads more successfully than they encoded the happy ones?

In my memory, anyhow, self-revulsion ads are the ones that haunt me most. Only now it's not just high-school acne I have to worry about. If that weren't bad enough, how disgusted would the pretty actress be by cancer, autoimmune disease, "grandma" hip surgery?

––––––

The type of unnecessary, stinging comment from the man in the elevator is one thing on its own, but the hurt is cumulative. The fear of being *even grosser than a pimple* builds and it builds and it builds.

At that moment in the elevator, I knew that my "deathyness" was showing. *Mortality* sounds like a more proper term, but what I mean here is slightly different. I'm not talking about the state of being subject to death, a state we all experience as humans. I mean the state of having some kind of palpable connection to it—the reminder that you can be young and yet seem, to some people, decrepit.

That small cloud of deathyness had started wafting around me two years earlier, when, in a series of unexpected moments, my body sent me into anaphylaxis, with no known cause. The coworker who saved my life by taking me down the block to the coincidentally nearby hospital watched my body fall into another place, then come back. "I feel like I'm talking to a ghost," he whispered the next day when he saw me emerge. He couldn't believe I was standing there and trying to talk about regular things to shake it off.

That's deathyness. Until specialists half figured out why my body was trying to kill itself, until I started coming to terms with the fact that I was a person who had almost died but was alive, I walked around a feeble, hollow version of myself. I was unable to really laugh or smile or know if my windpipe would swell again. I eventually tried to hang out with friends, but even though we were all recent college grads, I suddenly felt twice as old.

Talve-Goodman, despite sleeping with a guy who made her feel attractive and not like an oddity, writes in her essay about this same phenomenon. "I had waited nearly two years for a heart," she writes, "and, a year ago, I had come so close to death that sometimes I worry the smell of it lingers on my body and maybe that's the reason I buy so many clothes and creams."

Anne Thomas, a lawyer and a professional storyteller, writes of her feelings in a *New York Times* piece: "The prospect of romance is really the only thing that makes me think of myself as disabled."[25] With all the rude and ignorant comments people made about her use of a wheelchair, including telling her that her husband was a saint for marrying her, she began to absorb these ideas about herself. When she got married, she writes, even though she and her husband had a great life together, "I felt lucky, as if I had been pulled off the seconds shelf."

The way our culture demands that women be nubile and gyrating and luscious and fertile makes any hint of physical health issues—hint of moving toward death—a trigger for disgust. And just like in those old Bioré strip ads, the disgust that we learn to expect from others starts coming from ourselves, too.

On a blog called *Bitches Gotta Eat*, writer Samantha Irby posts about relationships and having Crohn's disease, among other experiences she mines for humor and sharp insights. In one post, her friend Cara calls her and says simply, "Black or fat?"[26]

Irby has no idea what her friend is talking about, but Cara keeps asking.

> "sam, you need to decide. BLACK or FAT?"
> "um, both i guess? no one's ever asked me to choose before.
> there's no fat box to check on the census."

Finally, Cara reminds Irby that they'd joked about going to a speed dating event. Cara is signing up to go and is trying to decide between the "chocolate singles mingle" and "curvy girls rule." At the prospect of either limiting herself to men of her own race or men who might be "losers hoping to take advantage of some low self-esteem" and body-image issues, Irby decides on the curvy event. But when Cara comes to her house all done up for speed dating, Irby is surprised. She realizes that the practical, "parent-teacher conference" pants she was going to wear aren't in the same league as her friend's outfit. She feels dirty standing next to her friend, even though she just showered: that old disgust we aim at ourselves. She tries to fix her hair—then starts having diarrhea. Which she's dealt with for twenty years, she writes, as someone with Crohn's disease. Here, though, it bumps up against her already insecure feelings about going to a speed dating event that she'd previously meant as a joke.

When Irby says she'll have to wear a diaper, Cara is unfazed and replies, "i have a bottle of perfume in my bag in case some shit leaks out, to cover up the smell." Irby writes about Cara's gesture:

> i love my fucking friends.
>
> so i put on one of my best bras, used a cotton ball to wipe A+D [diaper rash ointment] on my anus, slathered diaper cream in my butt, folded some soft gauze pads between my ass cheeks, pulled on a depends, and immediately started to panic. "i can't go," i blurted, on the verge of tears. "no one wants to date this person." i waved my hand at all of my butt supplies and accoutrement piled on the bathroom sink. "no dude wants to be with a broad who goes through 19 rolls of toilet paper in a month. I'm staying the fuck home." . . .
>
> i put my face paint on anyway, blubbering the whole time that i should just throw in the dating towel and wait until I'm fifty and can find some sixty-year-old who can actually relate to all of my incessant LEAKING.

She's getting at what a lot of young women have told me: their fear that most of the people they want to date can't relate or will be grossed out. She's getting at the reason I've sometimes wished for a partner who'd also been through hard things.

Irby and her friend do go to the speed dating night. Irby has a funny and possibly promising exchange with one guy. Then, she writes,

> it was my turn to laugh. and i did, pretty hard. and then i shit my diaper.
> what a betrayal this fucking body is.

A few years later, Irby ends up publishing a collection of essays based on her blog, and marrying a woman.[27]

Okay, I think, when I learn that last part: is it fair to consider how women like Irby and me do in relationships when we don't date men?

I put out a call for queer and transgender women dealing with serious health issues. A woman named Jen e-mails me. She introduces herself as a chronically ill, bisexual ethnic studies instructor.

"I've been in the medical complex from a very young age," she tells me. When she was born, she says, a lot of the muscles and tendons in her body were too short. She's had extensive surgeries: the first when she was about three years old, then the most major operations when she was eleven and twelve, and the latest when she was twenty-four. She still deals with the issues every day.

"I ended up with essentially the feet of an eighty-year-old by the time I was ten," she says, echoing many of the women I've met or read about who compare their bodies and, in a sense, their identities to someone decades older. At twenty-eight, Jen has been through a lot. She had all those surgeries for her muscles and tendons. She also has osteoarthritis, which started when she was a kid. Then, in junior high school, she had mental health issues that kept getting misdiagnosed. She was sent to a psychiatrist who gave her medicine that was dangerous for her—including one drug that hadn't been approved by the US Food and Drug Administration for adolescents and that landed her in the hospital for suicidal thoughts. More recently, she was diagnosed with fibromyalgia. She identifies as disabled—invisibly disabled. And although she's dated men and women, it's been the men who treated her differently once they found out she had issues with her joints and connective tissue.

There are the guys who've asked Jen if she can still have sex, and if she can, if she can have sex "normally." And then there was the guy in college whom she met on a blind date. The two of them clicked. She told him that she didn't want to have sex right away and that she'd experienced a certain amount of trauma going through these misdiagnoses and improper treatments for mental health issues when she'd been younger. Instead of listening, he tried to pressure her into having sex, even though she'd already said no.

Jen shut down. She cried. She tried to tell him again that she didn't want to have sex right away. The guy responded.

"I'm sorry, Jen," he said. "I should have realized that you're damaged."

———

At another point, Jen was in a longer-term relationship with a guy when she had one of her surgeries. For a while afterward, she had to use a cane. She noticed that the street harassment she got from older men now incorporated references to her mobility aid.

"Give me your cane," one man on the street said to her. "I know you don't really need it."

There were other moments. But one of the worst, she says, was when she walked down the street with her male partner. An older man, in reference to the cane, said, "What happened?"

"Actually, I was born this way," Jen said.

The street harasser responded, "Fuck you, bitch."

*Whaaat*, I hear myself saying to Jen, even though, when I think about it, she's just describing a more venomous version of interactions I've experienced before. It's a version of the man in the elevator who "corrected" the story of my crutches and told me how I should be presenting it instead. Understandably, in that moment on the street, Jen was upset. But her partner at the time, who was with her when it happened, told her that she should have responded to the man's question differently. That it was her fault, in fact, that the man said, "Fuck you, bitch."

"He said I should have [made up] some kind of story and that the guy was right to be mad at me," Jen tells me. "That I should have said something funny, because he was just trying to be funny."

To the guy she was in a relationship with, the street harasser's anger and venom were justifiable.

What about when she's dated women? I ask. Actually, it takes me an entire minute or two to ask about her experience, because I'm tripping over myself to not perpetuate preconceived notions of gender.

"Not to devolve into stereotypes," I say, "but I wonder . . . I'm wondering . . . when you've dated women . . . do you ever notice . . . I mean, not to say . . . of course, it's not that women are magically all wonderful, but I'm wondering . . . if there's a difference—"

"Big difference," Jen says, saving me from myself. "Yeah, there is a really obvious difference. When I was dating, and dating men and women, I found that there was a lot more tolerance and openness for difference when I was talking to women." So when she told women about her disability, she says, it was never much of an issue. "And there's something about queer people," she adds. As members of a group with queer bodies and an understanding of spectrums, queer people "have a much broader tolerance for liminality: for people being in kind of an in-between space."

She points out that in the academic world she's in, there's a big connection here. Indeed, queer studies and disability studies have been noticeably intersecting more at universities and in academic literature. Books like *Feminist, Queer, Crip* and *Crip Theory: Cultural Signs of Queerness and Disability* have appeared in recent years, and scholarship at these intersections has emerged at top schools.[28]

"My disability is so weird," Jen says, "because I don't look like a [person with a disability]." And yet, she does have one, even more than one.

"I'm struggling myself with using the word 'disability' or not," I tell her. We definitely have ideas about what counts as having a disability, and even though I have a bunch of serious health issues, chronic pain, joint surgery, and other illnesses, I'm just not sure these things amount to a disability, exactly.

Jen hears where I'm coming from and explains why the term makes sense to her.

"The reason why I decided to use this word," she says, was that it raises the question "Was the world designed with my body in mind? Can I access these spaces in the built environment and can I function in it healthily, or was my body not thought of when this institution was created?" For her, she says, "the answer is no, most of the time. But," she continues, "I'm also a fan of thinking of disability as something more liminal. I ask my students, if my campus was designed for people with wheelchairs, would they [still] be disabled?"

The understanding of being betwixt and between different spaces, she says, and even celebrating being between them, may be part of why dating fellow queer women was also so much easier with her health issues.

"Within heterosexual dating culture," she says, the men she's dated have thought "less about getting to know me as a person and more about what role I can perform in their life." It often felt that men were saying, "Prove to me that you're actually still a 'real woman.'"

Men she did date, she says, were often passive-aggressive, trying to get Jen to fit into their lives (something that women with and without disabilities can relate to throughout history). Jen lives in Colorado, where outdoorsy types abound, regardless of gender, and where many people focus on hiking, rock climbing, and other sports. But when she met women who weren't interested in dating her because she couldn't go out and do all the physical things the women were hoping for in a mate, the women were clear and up-front. They would just say flat-out that she and they might have different lifestyles and that it might not work. Even in these cases, she felt that women were more interested in her as a whole person. Those who brought up potential lifestyle conflicts were still open and affirming, she says, compared with most men she met, who often automatically viewed her as less sexually desirable, less fun, less of a perfect prop for the lives they had mapped out.

"I think there's also just a meta narrative about people with disabilities not being sexy or sexual," she says. "And so I've had a few instances where I've had men try to pressure me into doing sexual things before it is appropriate . . . as a way to prove that I'm still sexy." After she would disclose her health issues to them, she said, they would frame their pressuring her into sex as trying to get her to feel empowered. She can't tell, she says, if they think they can take advantage of a woman with a disability—a woman who might have low self-esteem—or if they really want to just see her prove that she's still desirable.

"I do definitely think that it has to do with the fact that my disability is invisible," she says. Her friends who use mobility aids like wheelchairs, she says, find that in the minds of the men they try dating, these friends "aren't even sexual at all—that isn't even on the table."

Jen's thoughts remind me of a piece I came across on *DapperQ*, a popular queer site that describes itself as "the premier queer style and empowerment website specifically for masculine-presenting women and trans-identified individuals." In a post called "Dapper Crip: Disability, Queer Masculinity, and Fashion," the folks being interviewed talk about "queercrip"—that intersecting space between queerness and disability. Jax Jacki Brown is pictured toward the top of the page. It's a powerful image, one that exudes sexuality: Jax in a wheelchair, photographed from behind, with close-cropped dyed-red hair and a tight black leather jacket. On the back of the jacket is a patch with white lettering. It reads *fuckability*. The chair itself has a decal on it, too. Brown describes the image: "a stick-figure wheelchair user being straddled by somebody."

For Jen, though, even with a more invisible disability, she has repeatedly come up against this idea of having to prove her fuckability, her sexual prowess.

Her current boyfriend, a guy she's been with for two years when we speak, sounds different from those she's dated before. She describes going with his family on a trip to China. When his mother was all go-go-go, Jen's boyfriend "was really conscientious," she says. He checked in with Jen privately to see what she needed, then told his mother if they needed to reevaluate the strenuousness of their next plans. While a conscientious partner does not magically undo the hurt that has come before, Jen's boyfriend seems to love her in a more holistic way—unlike the men who saw her as more of an object that may or may not fit their "needs."

———

On the queer women's blog *Autostraddle*, I read a Q&A with Tyler Vile, a "23-year-old [N]ative and Jewish queer trans woman with Cerebral Palsy."[29] Much of the article is about Vile's polyamory. She says she's currently dating two people, on top of some other more casual relationships. She travels a lot and seems to have friends all over the country.

About having cerebral palsy, she says, "I'm most people's introduction to loving someone with a visible physical disability. There's a cultural expectation that if you're dating a disabled person, you're their sole caretaker. I'm bucking that by having lots of friends and lovers and making sure none of them fall into a caretaker role."

Vile's words stand out to me: a young woman with a disability actively trying to prevent any one person in her life from feeling overly taxed. Her description both upends the stereotype of becoming a burden to others while also implying that there could be some truth to it—a pitfall she's trying to avoid. Throughout the piece, she seems like a young woman who celebrates community and finds a lot of joy in it. But while Vile herself as a queer and poly trans woman operates outside heteronormative culture, that culture is still what she, and all of us, grew up with. It's one that expects women to take on a caretaker role as mothers, wives, or girlfriends and expects men to be taken care of. What happens when a woman is the one who needs extra care from a partner or partners? Is that perhaps why those studies found that men were more likely to leave women with brain tumors than women were to leave men with the same condition? And given the spectrum of queer sexualities and gender identities, does it even make sense to ask these questions?

At a feminist bookstore-café in Bridgeport, Connecticut, I come across a slim and yellowing volume: *Voices from the Shadows: Women with Disabilities Speak Out*. The book looks both outdated and quite relevant, even though it's from 1983 and much has changed in the way we talk about disability, as well as women, in the intervening decades. Yet that's exactly why the pages draw me in. I want to see what, among all the changes in our discourse and thinking, has stayed the same.

The author, Gwyneth Ferguson Matthews, speaks with a retired psychotherapist named Dr. Brandt. For many years, the doctor had specialized in rehabilitation and is herself, like Matthews, a woman with quadriplegia, hers the result of childhood polio. On the whole, Matthews writes, Brandt thought that women with disabilities had an easier time integrating into society than did men with disabilities.

"However," Matthews writes, "she felt there was one area of exception: 'I think women have the disadvantage in dating and mating,'" Brandt tells her. "'I think it has always been the traditional role that women were the nurturing ones who took care of the helpless—children or wounded knights.'" And so, the psychiatrist tells Matthews, she suspects that men with disabilities probably get married more than their female counterparts do.[30]

And what about queer relationships? Surely, women have left women who got sick. But again, from all I was hearing, it wasn't very common. As Audre Lorde writes in *The Cancer Journals*, "A lifetime of loving women had taught me that when women love each other, physical change does not alter that love. It did not occur to me that anyone who really loved me would love me any less because I had one breast instead of two, although it did occur to me to wonder if they would be able to love and deal with the new me."[31] Here, Lorde means something deeper than her physical appearance.

As Simon and I grew closer, moved in together, spent time with each other's families, got domestically partnered, helped each other with work projects, traveled all over together, I kept thinking there would be a tipping point. You're just too medically fucked up, I'd imagine him saying. After all, my health issues kept getting in the way. On a trip to Japan, we had to skip an entire city because my joint pain was severe. Then we had to spend an entire afternoon in Singapore, our next stop, trying to find a doctor who could help. I felt like a burden. Simon showed that we were in it together, standing in a tropical downpour, waiting for the deluge to stop so we could cross the street to the hospital. He didn't mind. In fact, even that day, with me in pain and our plans revolving around hospital hours, we had fun, laughing in the rain, entertaining each other as we waited. He showed me that love could still feel sparkly and magical and all those things we hope for in a relationship, regardless of a messed-up ankle or hip or thyroid or flap. Because he is not like that man in the elevator who told me to just pretend it was my knee, Simon helped me see that an onslaught of health issues didn't have to affect attraction or love.

Eventually, I started to believe him. That so-in-love feeling of walking around holding hands at night, or kissing when no one's looking, or sending each other clever puns? Maybe it wouldn't actually get punctured by my doctors' appointments or the tinctures that specialists made me try or the way I sometimes felt more sick than young.

I'd love to say that I created my feelings of self-worth all on my own in an Oprah-approved vacuum of celestial empowerment. The reality is that Simon, an external force, a person outside of myself, helped. And it's not that he was some perfect, otherworldly creature, either (though sometimes he seemed that way, and still does). We'd had difficult relationship issues to work out, and both of us were, like all humans, flawed. But when it came to my health, he never batted an eye. He never made me feel as if I had to live up to some sexist idea of what a woman is supposed to be. Sometimes we joked that because I was a woman, and white, and he was a man, and black, we each came to the relationship with different sets of privilege and different daily prejudices flung at us, and maybe these experiences helped us at least *try* to see past the stereotypes the other had to contend with.

Reading a piece in the *New York Times* about a breeding program for endangered penguins, I happen upon a passage that feels personal. The piece describes two "star-crossed lovers." There's Guinn, a male with "prized genes," and Jumoke, "whose genetic makeup is less optimal," though Guinn "doesn't much care about that."[32]

What does "less optimal" mean in terms of genetics? It makes me a bit upset, but I immediately relate to Jumoke.

The piece goes on. While an animal keeper says the science center has assigned Guinn to a different mate for breeding purposes, "he keeps coming back to Jumoke." Guinn, the *Times* reports, "would serve the species by moving on, of course, but he just can't quit her."

Maybe, I think, it's because he can't detect her "less optimal" genes the way the humans breeding the birds can. Or maybe I should just be heartened that these penguins, regardless of health, are still in love and don't subscribe to our eugenics-tinged ideas.

The only remarks Simon makes about my health are affectionate: "You're like a riot wrapped in skin," he says one day, when he sees how much I'm going through with a newer diagnosis. It's clear that he means it like this: I love that riot.

When, five years into my partnership with Simon, I realized, slowly and then rapidly, that I might be gay and needed to date women, he was as loving as ever. The realization was at times excruciating for both of us, but he offered me the space to try it out.

The woman I started dating, Bailey, wasn't scandalized in the least by my newly open relationship with Simon—or, luckily, by my health history, which I revealed faster to her than I had with others, though still not all at once.

One day, when Bailey and I were at her apartment and heading out to buy some groceries, she made a comment that's usually hard for me to navigate.

"Your bag looks heavy," she said. "You can just leave it here—the grocery store's right down the block."

"Oh, it's cool. I'll just take it with me," I said, trying to play it all casual, when really the only reason I take my tote bag everywhere is that my EpiPens don't fit in my pocket.

"Okay. We're really just going two blocks away, though. You just need your wallet," she said, just as people before her had said for years: lovers, friends who were just getting to know me, the well-meaning brother of someone I had dated. But unlike those other times, I decided to just come out with it.

"Uh, it's actually 'cause I carry emergency medicine, and it doesn't fit in my pocket," I said. I hoped it didn't freak her out. For folks with clunkily shaped health paraphernalia, a minor thing like a tote bag suddenly matters. "I have never had a purse that wasn't wide enough for an EpiPen, deep enough for an inhaler, and complete with a zippered pocket for Benadryl," the poet Sandra Beasley writes.[33] Bags can become a question of how much to reveal.

But Bailey was not surprised by a young person who'd gotten close to her mortality. When she was just twelve years old, she had watched a friend go through an awful cancer. She'd sat with her in the hospital room, unsure if her friend would survive. The friend did survive, luckily, but went through years of chemotherapy and uncertainty. Right after that experience, Bailey had watched another classmate go through the same thing. This time, the boy died. And although Bailey hadn't had the extreme medical conditions I had, she had a body that tended toward my end of the spectrum: several chronic health issues that she dealt with weekly or daily and that one might not expect in someone her age.

"I wish I weren't so *delicate*," she'd say, enunciating the final word like a curse. We talked about how being so damn delicate didn't fit with our concept of ourselves, our sporty childhoods, our independence and pride.

Bailey was only twenty-seven when we met, and I, thirty-one. We agreed that those numbers didn't quite capture the moments of mortality we'd been through or witnessed. We both found it a relief to date someone who understood the tension between being an active person and having a body with painful joints or inconvenient reactions. At the same time, I thought, this shared understanding could have drawbacks, too. If two people who'd grown to love each other wanted to help each other through health issues, what to do if they both had flare-ups at the exact same time? And was there a point at which it became psychologically unhealthy to sit around talking about the times deathyness had entered your young life?

I wasn't sure which was worse: feeling like a burden to a partner who had her or his own health issues to deal with or feeling like a burden to a partner who couldn't relate. Something about Bailey's having a body and gender experience closer to mine did make me less worried for a while. Less vulnerable, more automatically accepted for my differences, as Jen, who's bi, had said was her experience, too. But for all of my overlap with Bailey, I'd still internalized the airbrushed cultural images my whole life. And I'd heard about all these women who'd been ditched. By men, yes, but that didn't wholly quell my fears.

One day, after I'd developed a small but visible syndrome that was making me feel unattractive—something that my doctor said often goes away in a year or two but that caused my eyelids to swell in my sleep once or twice a week—I started to cry. It felt petty, to have lived through cancer and my throat closing up and all this surgery and then to cry about how my eyelid skin was getting slightly stretched out from the repeated swelling, but I found myself sobbing. And I heard myself saying out loud to Bailey things that I hadn't even realized were in me. "Will you still find me attractive if one of my eyelids gets slightly droopy?" I asked. "One already has a tiny fold from the swelling. What if my eyes don't look as symmetrical anymore? What if in five months I get more weird lines around my eyes and you're like, *Meh?*"

All our similarities in terms of gender and deathyness still didn't mean, I realized, that we had the same things happening. This wasn't like getting food poisoning as a couple. Bailey's eyes were fine.

And with Simon, with whom I had fewer body overlaps, I felt pretty safe from rejection—more because we had developed so much love, trust, and commitment over the years. But I didn't feel completely safe from it. Simon, the most incredible partner I could hope for, someone who made every day burst with happiness and adventure, comfort and warmth, was still the healthy one to my sick. No matter how much he showed me that he loved me regardless of my body and immune system, I still, in the back of my mind, wondered if he'd become repelled: by my medicine, by my hip joints, by the meaning of the scar that still spread faintly across my neck.

# PART 2

# The (Foggy) Glass Ceiling and the Wall

At my first job out of college, I didn't grasp the point of human resources. I was twenty-one, and although I'd had one hip surgery already, none of my other health issues had struck. I didn't think much about the reasons that someone might need to take off from work. And *human resources* sounded suspiciously like something out of *Soylent Green*, or maybe Orwell. Even if it didn't remind me of dystopian meals made of people, did we really need an entire team whose sole role, it seemed, was to make formal job offers to you over the phone so that your soon-to-be boss wouldn't have to feel awkward telling you how little you were worth in US currency?

My job started: legal assistant to the associate general counsel of an international nonprofit. My title, I learned, really meant I'd be working as hard as an attorney, just without the degree. The position required a ton of training and learning, and although I was also writing at night and trying to publish my work, the nonprofit work in the day was taking up most of my hours and energy.

One afternoon in the office, a wild, prickly, hot feeling rose from my ears. And then my face swelled. I didn't know why.

"Uh, are you okay?" my coworker Michael asked. He was a few years older than I was and we were starting to be friends.

"Yeah, I just have, I dunno—my face just got swollen for some reason."

"You're having an allergic reaction," Michael said.

"But I'm not allergic to anything."

"Your face is out to here." He held his hands half a foot from both cheeks. "I'm taking you to the hospital."

The hospital, luckily, was on our block. It just so happened to be a short walk. When we got to the emergency room, Michael helped me sign in. And suddenly I had to go to the bathroom. After the person at the front desk pointed to the restroom, I went inside and peed.

And then, as I turned the handle to open the bathroom door, everything went black.

When I opened my eyes, I was on the floor screaming. All kinds of strangers were standing over me, shouting things, lifting me, containing me, carting me across the room as I flailed. I couldn't see or hear or breathe the way I was used to seeing and hearing and breathing. A type of pain that I'd never felt before and never felt again zapped every millimeter of every organ and membrane inside me, making me thrash about, while at the same time my whole self began to dim.

A needle plunged into some part of me. More shouts. Then a sudden corkscrew feeling, as if my entire body were being pulled from underwater at ninety miles an hour in a spiral, as if some wave or gust were sucking me into tiny rapid circles while lifting me up, up, up.

*Did you eat nuts? Are you allergic to nuts? Do you know how dangerous this is?* I remember one doctor hurling these questions at me. He looked terrified.

Once my senses roared back to life, I could see the room around me. Michael was gone, but now my mother was there, looking terrified. I didn't know how much time had elapsed. I still don't know what happened in between.

The epinephrine injection probably caused the surreal feeling that my body was being sucked upward in a corkscrew pattern and then deposited back to earth and this emergency room, though I've still never asked a doctor why that particular feeling might have occurred. And I'd seen no white light, none of that stuff people see. But I had come within a few seconds of no longer being alive.

––––

The emergency room in Manhattan had saved my life, no question about it, and, really, my coworker Michael had saved it first by dragging me there. After the doctors had kept me overnight to monitor me, I woke up exuberant, with medicine perhaps still coursing through me. When a doctor came in to check on me, I told him what I'd just remembered. I know this sounds funny, I said, but today is the day I'm supposed to fly to India to visit a friend.

And so, because I had bought the tickets months earlier and was hopped up on life-reviving chemicals and because the doctors weren't even sure what had caused my reaction—and because I was used to living in a body that usually worked well, was twenty-two years old, and generally didn't die—I did what now seems completely unreasonable. I packed a suitcase and flew to Kolkata.

Once there, I told my friend Smita what had happened in the emergency room. It sounded unreal to her and to me. Like a fluke. So it didn't stop us from boarding a train from Kolkata to Darjeeling to visit the tea plantations her grandmother thought we should see.

In the train station, I felt dizzy. Maybe I was just exhausted from the whole body-shutting-down thing and then immediately flying halfway across the globe. I ate a banana.

After thirty minutes on the train, maybe forty, the seats and faces around me got hazy. Everything moved slowly; everything got dim.

"Uh, Smita," I said. "I don't wanna scare you, but I think it's happening again. I think I'm gonna pass out."

My blood pressure was dropping, and my vision was starting to tunnel, but I heard Smita ask if there was a doctor onboard. Then, somehow, she got the express train to make an emergency stop. She held my hand to help me off the train and onto the road, hailed us an auto-rickshaw, and tried to keep me awake.

I spent six days in the hospital and got weaker before I recovered. Or, I wasn't sure what it meant to recover. Later in the week, a nurse took my blood pressure, looked at Smita, and shook her head. "Very low," she whispered. She wasn't sure how my body would get back across the ocean to New York.

And this is where human resources comes in. I needed it. A lot. In the slivers of minutes when I remembered things beyond how to stay conscious, I realized I couldn't go back to work. This big vacation to India was my first time taking two weeks off from my new job, a job I'd been at for only about five months. My image of human resources—of happily employed people who lazed about and handed out folders—immediately shifted once I realized how much time I'd need to take off and how much I was at the mercy of my office.

But then, at some point, there came the reassuring voice of an HR person on the phone, telling me that everyone realized how awful this was, that Michael had seen me near death, that the whole department understood that health comes first, and that I had some options. My colleague in HR told me about the Family and Medical Leave Act and explained the options I had (either take the leave or take sick days) so soothingly that I stopped worrying that my suddenly unreliable health might jeopardize my job. My coworkers called me to ask how I was feeling. After a scary trip back to the United States by myself, unable to walk on my own, and unsure of what would happen on the plane, I took a week of sick days at my parents' house and tried to regain my strength. My office mates called again to check in on me and to tell me to take as long as I needed. I was embarrassed that my coworker Michael had seen me lose control of my body. But I knew, too, that when he saw the need to whisk me out of the office and into the hospital, he had also saved that body's life.

I was starting to feel like a much older person, a person trying to just have fun and start my career but who kept tripping over an unusual amount of shit. My one-checkup-a-year interaction with doctors turned into several appointments every few weeks. I learned that I had a rare condition called idiopathic anaphylaxis, or mast-cell activation syndrome, a life-threatening allergic reaction whose cause was unknown. I spent every day unsure whether my throat would close up again.

Three years went by. And then, at a new office, I learned what happens when the people you work with forget that you're human, not just a work machine. (And forget that a human, even a young human, is an assortment of cells that do their own thing when you're not looking.)

After I'd been working as an intern at a magazine for a few months, my boss told me that my writing and editing stood out. And—dream of intern dreams—she wanted to hire me full-time. I said yes to the offer and to a start date in the fall, even though I knew the magazine was trying to save money by keeping me an unpaid intern for longer than they should have before my new position started. So I kept working for free, until the official day when my title kicked in and I moved to the staff side of the office.

On my first day, I was raring to go as a real-life staff editor, ready to keep working hard as part of the staff. But that evening, I had a doctor's appointment right at the end of the workday—an appointment I had been putting off. It was the last installment in a series of less and less fun occasions. Months earlier, I'd been in a checkup with my regular doctor. She had palpated my neck—what a gross, gross word, I thought, *palpate*, those *p*'s that make popping noises on radio interviews when the mic work isn't stellar, and that *-pate*, like a scalp. My doctor had moved her hands over my lymph nodes and felt a tiny lump.

Everyone knows it: a lump is often not good. Then I had an imaging test. I spotted the lump and its little frightening friend, lump number two, on the screen, tilting my head in a way that the technician did not appreciate. But I had to see it. I had to know that it was really there. "Oh god, those look bad, right?" I asked. The technician looked half at what she was doing with the ultrasound on my neck and half at the screen, trying not, it seemed, to really see. "You'll get the results in a few days after the radiologist reads them," she said curtly. "But, right," I said, "I mean, it looks bad, right?" I couldn't stop saying it, prepping myself for the worst. She conceded, somehow. I don't remember what she said, but she acknowledged with her eyebrows that it might be bad, yes.

After that, I'd had what's called a fine needle aspiration—a long, painful needle in my neck to get a biopsy of my thyroid. And then I had to wait until my doctor received the results.

Now it was the evening of my first day as an official, paid, full-time staff member of this magazine I'd interned for since the summer, and I was at my doctor's office. And the results were bad.

"You have papillary thyroid cancer," my doctor said, reading off the chart instead of really looking at me, or at least that's how I remember it. A lot of interactions with medical clinicians seemed to be them giving awful news while trying to avert their eyes.

Then, a mess of sadness and anger. I'd need surgery, maybe further treatment. After calling a few friends and getting myself back to my apartment to confront this newest of unexpected, awful news, I realized I had to tell my boss. But I'd first need a day to process things. I could barely register that I had cancer, barely picture myself telling my own mother what I'd been diagnosed with. I e-mailed my boss, the woman who'd known me for months when I was an intern, and told her I wasn't feeling well and would need the day off. I said I would also need to meet with her about something important: something that I'd like her to keep private. I copied my more immediate supervisor on the message, as I sensed from my internship that my boss was not always the warmest.

I'm not sure what I did on that sick day, other than sit around in my pajamas and think about the word *tumor*. One day to process it, to let the shock run through me. And then, the next day, I went back to work.

"I hope there's a good reason you were out yesterday," my boss said. She was walking past my desk, which is to say she was walking past everyone's desk, as our cubicles were all scrunched together in a row. Everyone could hear what she was saying, the growl of it.

"There is, and . . . I'll explain it later when we meet?" I didn't mean to sound meek, but I did.

"Good," she said. She looked pissed. "Because I need to be able to explain to Ted"—the magazine's temperamental overlord—"why you missed your second day of work."

I wanted to tell her that it was a very good reason and that, anyway, didn't she get to know me all those months during my internship and hire me because she trusted me and my work ethic and my work? There was nothing to say, though. We had our weekly meeting with the whole staff later that morning, and I felt clammy just thinking about my boss's severe tone. How was I supposed to reconcile it with the fact of having cancer inside me?

"Michele," my boss said loudly while the entire staff was still shuffling out of the meeting. "You had something you wanted to talk to me about."

Yes, I thought, and yet again, had she missed the part where I said it was private?

A few of my colleagues lingered at the door for a moment to see what was happening. One friendly editor turned back, looking a bit intrigued, perhaps to see if I was okay. I tried to match my boss's loudness with my own uncharacteristic quietness, but of course, that makes people's ears perk up, too.

I told her that yes, I needed to talk with her, and gestured for my immediate supervisor to stay in the room as well. We sat at the big wooden conference table. I told them that the reason I'd needed to take yesterday off was that I learned the night before that I had cancer.

My eyes got all blurry, and I waited for the reply. My immediate editor, the colleague I'd asked to join the meeting as a kind of barrier between me and my boss, looked at me and said something warm and thoughtful. She looked pained, looking at me looking pained.

Our boss, meanwhile, led with a series of questions and blank stares. She asked if I was okay on health insurance, since they had only put me on payroll that week. Her tone, though, was less like "Oof, I'm sorry you have cancer. What are the next steps?" and more like, "You've got to be fucking kidding me."

"Uh, I hope you don't think I was hiding this," I said. "I really just found out two nights ago. I know it's bad timing that I found out my very first day on staff. I mean, I wouldn't have hidden it. . . . I mean, I guess, legally, I would have been allowed to not tell you when you hired me, but I didn't know, I really didn't know . . ." It sounded a lot like that, me stammering in the face of zero empathy.

"I need you to leave your cancer at the door," she said. "When you come in to the office in the morning, I need you to be here working. I don't want to hear about your cancer."

My boss stood up and shoved her chair against the table.

"Are we done here," she said.

It wasn't a question.

Over the next few weeks, there were several more moments in the office that felt off. But my brain was trying to figure out doctors' appointments so that I could meet various surgeons who might end up being the one who'd slice open my neck. And I was so busy trying to figure out how exactly to "leave my cancer at the door" that I didn't quite grasp in the moment how devoid of empathy my boss had been.

One thing that I did vaguely realize: the magazine had no human resources department. Or even one single human resources person. Nothing. And I thought of how the wonderful HR woman at my old job had made sure to convey that my illness was not a burden and not my fault.

Although I'd come into my first office role with the idea that the department was a bit of a joke, I had by now been through one medical emergency with HR and another without. And there was a palpable difference.

So I started to wonder. There seem to be plenty of people with stories about how HR failed them: during times of medical need, or sexual harassment, or layoffs. But how many workplaces across the United States simply don't have HR to begin with? And how does that affect people who get sick? Was I covered by the Americans with Disabilities Act? Did my boss break the law by terrorizing me about my cancer, or did she simply break a code of kindness and human decency?

———

A study on how rheumatic diseases affect people's vocations describes an important gender discrepancy: "Research suggests that women with disabilities typically experience higher unemployment rates than men with disabilities."[1]

And a 2015 study in the journal *Cancer* tracked more than seven hundred early-stage breast cancer patients (all of them women) to see how both the cancer and, for those who had it, the chemotherapy may have affected their employment. The study asked how the women were faring in the workplace four years after their diagnosis. Almost a third were out of work. And for those who'd undergone chemotherapy, 38 percent were unemployed.[2]

Meanwhile, even women who stay employed while dealing with medical issues must grapple with a lot. While not everyone's boss is as nightmarish as my old boss had been when I had cancer, there are plenty of other awkward moments with colleagues, supervisors, or professors and worries that even working hard at one's career won't be enough to compensate for illness. Especially if your career is just beginning.

Take Karen, a young woman who identifies as white, straight, and Jewish. She began having strange stomach pains soon after starting law school. She was at Harvard. She was throwing up a lot, nauseous all the time, and losing weight without knowing why. The student health center told her she was a little anemic. The medical staff told her to take some iron. They told her to take antacids. For a year and a half, she could barely keep food down.

In her second year of law school, she had such extreme abdominal pain, she thought she had appendicitis. She went to the hospital and learned that not only was her appendix inflamed, but so were her intestines. She had a colonoscopy and then, finally, received a diagnosis: severe Crohn's disease.

When the medication she received for her Crohn's didn't work, she was back in the hospital for a week. And then, back again. An infection had formed an abscess the size of a soda can outside her intestines, and she had to get it drained. At some point, she realized the severity of the condition. She would have to take a leave of absence from school—and she would have to cancel her summer associate job.

Harvard law students are competitive about their summer jobs—ones that many law students consider a necessary stepping-stone to the full-time job they want after graduation. The firm they work at the summer after their second year as a summer associate is often the place they hope will hire them once they get their degree a year later. And, Karen says, the program is fun. Not only was she formally withdrawing from school for a semester and moving back to her parents' house in Maine, but she would miss out on the summer job that she was really looking forward to.

She was only just starting her career, and now she felt derailed.

After her semester off and a summer spent dealing with doctors instead of working, Karen found that being back at school wasn't the same. She felt as if she were in a shell, she says, because she just didn't want to tell any of her professors about her health issues. And she didn't want to share her situation with any classmates who didn't already know. Crohn's disease is a very embarrassing disease, she says, and there are many misconceptions about it. For one, it has to do with going to the bathroom: embarrassing. And people think Crohn's is the same as irritable bowel syndrome, she says, which is something different. People also think you can change your diet and be fine. Adding to her challenges, Karen's type of Crohn's is a less common manifestation of the disease. It affects her upper gastrointestinal tract, not her lower. She didn't want to have to explain it to people over and over again. "No, I don't have the kind where I'm pooping all the time," she found herself saying, "but I do have Crohn's, and it's very serious."

Taking a leave of absence, she says, felt like showing weakness. She was afraid people wouldn't want to work with her or wouldn't want her opinion. She thought that a tougher person would have just powered through, even if, in her case, powering through wasn't really possible.

People will think less of me, she thought. They wouldn't value my work as much if they knew I had a disability.

Now, after getting through the rest of school, Karen works at a law firm where the workload and expectations are so heavy that some of her colleagues sleep in the office. "I just really can't do that," she says. "I know that there's a direct correlation between lack of sleep and stress and my Crohn's and my lupus"—a second autoimmune disease that Karen developed from her Crohn's medication.

Knowing that her health issues mean she can't stay all night in the office, Karen finds that she's become more efficient. She plans ahead. She doesn't wait till the last minute when there's a deadline. Still, she says, others' work hours have an effect. "If the person in charge stays all night, you're expected to, too."

"I haven't had a performance review yet," she says, "but I feel like at my performance review, it might be mentioned that, you know, 'You're not a team player. You go home.' I mean, I can't see anyone saying, 'You go home at eleven p.m., tsk, tsk, tsk.' But, you know, the people on my team, they might want an explanation for why I'm not staying all night, too."

Some people at the firm do know about her Crohn's, but they are mainly the junior-level people. She hasn't told any of the partners, the higher-ups.

"It's weird because they have a legal obligation and I'm sure an ethical obligation to accommodate individuals with disabilities," she says. "But at the same time, it's a very high-pressure environment."

And there are awkward moments, moments where Karen isn't sure if she's accidentally outed herself to those in charge. While working on a pharmaceutical case, she and her colleagues started talking about medications. Her boss explained that the company they were dealing with makes biologics, and that it's okay if the team didn't know what kind of medicine that was. When Karen volunteered that she did know, her boss said, "Oh, did you get a medical degree, too?"

Karen forced a laugh, but she could tell her boss really did want to know where her knowledge came from. She kept laughing it off, but felt very, very awkward. This was a senior person. None of the other people in the meeting knew about her medical conditions, either.

———

I speak with Caryl Rivers, a journalism professor, and Rosalind C. Barnett, a senior scientist at the Women's Studies Research Center at Brandeis University who specializes in gender and workplace research. Rivers and Barnett have authored a number of books together, including *The New Soft War on Women: How the Myth of Female Ascendance Is Hurting Women, Men—and Our Economy.*

"Research shows that women have more mentors—people who will be nice to you," Rivers and Barnett tell me, "but men have more *sponsors*"—people who will really help you, speak up for you, and help you climb the ladder at work. Sponsors, Rivers and Barnett tell me, are the people who talk you up to the rest of your workplace.

They help establish you as an important member of the team. If you're experiencing a setback, like needing to take time off for cancer treatment, sponsors would make sure the rest of the office knows when you're back and that you're just as good as ever. Without sponsors, however, nobody has established your credibility as a hard or ingenious worker, and you may return from a medical issue without anyone there to back you up as a team member. As the authors write in *The New Soft War on Women*, "You and your male colleague may both have a mentor, but he'll get a sponsor—an advocate who will go to bat for him in a way that a woman's champion will not." And, they add, "you'll get more scrutiny than he will."[3]

In Karen's case at the law firm and in my case at the magazine, we're in offices and have salaries. Although the specter of being let go for reasons related to our health issues is a serious one—and although, without an HR person to mediate, I found myself negotiating sick days directly with my boss in awkward ways—our experiences are probably stable compared with young women with hourly jobs: retail, food service, and other service work.

I reach out to New York City's Paid Sick Leave Initiative, a relatively new campaign to enforce protections for workers, including those with hourly jobs. The initiative's representative tells me that until someone files a complaint against an employer, the story doesn't reach the city agency, meaning that there are many instances of employer discrimination that nobody at the agency hears about. That said, she gives me an example. A woman named Rosario worked as a supervisor at a coffee shop. She requested time off for a medical procedure related to brain surgery she'd had a few months before. But when she returned to work, her employer didn't pay for her sick leave. So the city agency investigated. It found that that Rosario's workplace not only failed to pay her for using properly accrued sick time but also failed to maintain a written sick leave policy and failed, too, to provide employees with the "Notice of Employee Rights." The parties agreed on a settlement, including $1,225 in civil penalties for the employer and more than $600 in restitution for Rosario. The agency also took steps to make sure that the café started to comply with the city's paid sick leave law.

But there are lots of people like Rosario who don't have any paid sick time off in the first place, who never get their lost wages back, or who find that their surgery or health condition jeopardizes a job that already pays very little. I ask a cofounder of a group called OUR Walmart, which advocates for the rights of Walmart associates, if he's heard any stories from young women being disrespected at work while dealing with health issues or disabilities. He certainly has. It's "a huge issue for Walmart workers," he replies. He connects me with a couple of women employed by the store—the largest retailer in the country. One of them is Brit, a woman who started at Walmart when she was about thirty-seven in a town she calls "the meth capital."

"I had cancer when I was four," Brit tells me. As we talk, I can hear her own five-year-old's voice over the phone. "Miracle baby," Brit calls him: after grueling cancer treatments when she was a kid, she didn't think she'd be able to have a child herself. The treatments wreaked havoc on her in other ways, too. When she was fifteen, she began to have kidney trouble in the form of chronic IgA nephropathy. In this condition, antibodies gather in the kidneys and cause inflammation. The cancer drugs also affected her joints. Now she wears a brace that goes up around her right calf, since her ankle locks if she stands still for too long.

A few months after Walmart hired her as a traditional checkout cashier, Brit realized that standing in one place for an entire shift was proving painful, even with her brace. She needed an assignment that let her move her legs a bit. Her doctor wrote a note explaining that she needed accommodation, and said that managing the self-checkout area would be ideal, since she would be able to walk between the eight registers to help customers and therefore keep her joints from getting stiff. Walmart said no. The store could switch her department altogether but wanted to keep the self-checkout area open to various employees to train. So her managers put her on light duty.

Then one day, a pair of boys were play-fighting in the store. One of them jumped and landed on Brit's toe. Having broken her toes before, she knew something in her foot was broken. And it hurt. One of her colleagues saw her and told her she looked ghastly. Brit replied that she felt like she was about to throw up. After a long while, they finally flagged down a manager. Brit clocked out and drove herself to the hospital, where an X-ray showed the break. The doctors told her to stay off her foot for the next three days and put her on pain medication. The next day, someone drove her to the store so that she could show her managers the note from the emergency room. "But ever since that moment," she says, "ever since I broke my toe, it's been totally downhill."

At some point, the store decided to have her fill out an accident report. Walmart had her go to a workers' comp doctor, who told her it was "just a contusion," despite the hospital X-rays showing otherwise. Walmart had her do tasks that weren't suitable for someone with a broken toe and someone who already had a known history of arthritis and joint issues. Unlike when she'd broken toes at other points in her life and they'd healed back up, this one never did. After continuing to walk on the injury that Walmart didn't take seriously enough, she had to take medical leave to allow it to heal. And then, when she came back from leave, she says, her supervisors suddenly gave her an attitude. But she kept working and even got the position she'd wanted at the self-checkout area. Then, things got worse again.

When Brit was in the shower one morning, she fell. She'd blacked out—for no discernable reason. Her husband got her dressed and took her to the emergency room, where the staff discovered several brain tumors. They were noncancerous but still caused symptoms, including excruciating migraines. Brit let her supervisors at work know.

"When I told them I found out I had noncancerous brain tumors," she says, "I wanted [them] to go, 'Well, let us help you to help us.'" She wanted them to offer a setup that would allow her to keep contributing to the team at work. Instead, she says, "it's like they've been trying to get rid of me."

Investigative journalists, watchdog nonprofits, and other concerned groups have long documented the problematic conditions at Walmart stores across the country. Often, the reports are of the store firing workers who the retailer believes are attempting to organize. In Brit's case, she was just trying to be treated with empathy while still keeping up with her shifts. She describes a few moments when things have gotten out of hand. One of her immediate supervisors, who used to be friendly to her but who started to be sharp after Brit's health issues, began to shout at Brit across the registers. The person supervising both of them called them into his office.

"I'm thirty minutes behind on my lunch, and I have a headache and don't want to be yelled at," Brit said.

"You need to leave your personal issues and your medical issues at home," the manager snapped back.

"I left his office crying," Brit tells me. "It was really bad."

"I had a boss at my old job say almost the same exact thing to me," I tell her.

"I take it from customers all day," she says. "I've been called racist, I've been called white trash, I've been called the C-word a couple of times. . . . I don't need it from managers."

"I was out of work for three months, and I had no money," Brit says of her medical leave. "I barely, barely survived. Thank god my husband had a job at the time and that my family owns the house we live in, or we would probably be on the street."

———

After Katherine Russell Rich found a lump in her breast at age thirty-two, her colleagues stopped seeing her as competent. In an essay for the *Washington Post*, she recalls a scene in which her own boss is perhaps more searingly forthright than mine was.[4]

"Sit down," her editor says at the start of her year-end evaluation. At this point in her cancer treatment, Rich writes, "the scarves were off. I looked like a Chia pet sprouting fiber optics, no pigmentation." Her boss speaks.

"I can't review your work," he says. "You haven't done much this year. I haven't wanted to give you things to do. Partly for humanitarian reasons. But partly because I wanted to be sure that they got done."

Rich assures him that they would have gotten done. That he could start giving her work to do now.

"You know," he chortles. "I really felt bad for you. No one here wanted anything to do with you because you reminded them they could die."

"He beamed," Rich writes, "like I was finally in on the joke. On the way out, a buzz in my head made me dizzy as embarrassment gave way to fear. The editor had fired people for lighter infractions than being walking reminders of death."

And there it is, that deathyness again. Rich's editor admitting that the whole office saw her as a reminder of their mortality, that no one wanted anything to do with her.

As the *New York Times* writes, Rich eventually was fired by one of her bosses, "apparently discomforted by Ms. Rich's cancer."[5] Put less passively, a human fired another human from a job she was good at. Fired her because she was sick.

The *Times* quote is from 2012. It's in an obituary for Rich. Something in me doesn't want to say that word, *obituary*. It's irrelevant, part of me thinks. She died so many years after her boss told her she was a walking reminder of death that it shouldn't lend any credence to his awful remark. Either way, what he did sounds potentially illegal.

But this is where our cultural ideas of efficiency and being an able worker surface in me. Why do I want to hide the part of the story where Rich eventually dies of cancer? Do I think no one will see the horror in what her boss said to her, once the reader knows that eventually she does die?

In the end, I want to be honest. Rich died of cancer in 2012. She was fifty-six. That doesn't mean her boss, twenty-four years earlier, when she was thirty-two, had license to say such hurtful things to her, presumably because he was uncomfortable around bodies that reminded him that he, too, would eventually die. Nor does it mean that if Rich had died that very same year, at thirty-two, her boss would have been free to say hurtful things, either.

When my boss said I'd need to "leave my cancer at the door," how much of her attitude was her own very human fear of death or reminders of death? And how much was her anger that she'd hired an intern to become a staff member, and now that staff member needed surgery and might not work at top speed for a few weeks?

I remember working extra, extra hard to prove that I could do as much quality work as anyone else could, cancer or not. I said yes to assignments that, logically, I wouldn't be able to do while in the hospital, all because my boss had put the fear of dismissal in me. If any trace of my cancer treatment came up at the office, if I had to say no to doing a story because I needed a few days to recover from surgery, then I might be seen as a worthless investment.

As if to test me when I'd returned from my thyroid surgery, my boss added an entirely new set of requirements to my job. I had been hired as an editor, which, at this magazine, meant that I'd be both editing and writing articles for the print magazine. Now, my boss said, I would also be creating the package of stories on the home page, coming up with a new combination of text, images, and headlines and five to ten articles every day to constitute the face of the magazine online. The content management system was notorious for crashing, so creating anything online was a mess. I knew this would mean late nights for me. Late nights and a headache that nobody else in the office would have, because suddenly this was my job, when before it had been the shared domain of the interns, a burden distributed across several people.

*Huh, I don't think this whole new thing was in my job description when you hired me,* I wanted to say. I might have said it, had I not had the cancer to compensate for. "Ohh, uh, okay," I said instead, trying to look casual about an enormous increase in my set of responsibilities, knowing that one whiff of a medical reason for not wanting to add an entirely new facet to an already-demanding position might get me fired. There seemed to be something cruel and not quite kosher about dropping a new set of responsibilities on me that hadn't been discussed previously, and dropping it right as my body was recovering from cancer.

But then, it's only in hindsight that I see the cruelty and strangeness of it. At the time, I just had fear. I feared betraying any sign of my illness to my boss—I cringed when I had to tell her that I'd need an extra hour at lunch to go to my post-surgical checkup, but there was no way around it when the surgeon's hours were only during the workday—and I feared that my boss would look at me one day and say, *Aha! See! Your cancer made you a bad employee!* So I worked harder than I should have for what I was paid for, harder than I should have for what my body was going through, harder than I might have without any health issues, to show that I was worthwhile, like everyone else.

Sometimes, though, a person gets struck by a health problem that will in fact interfere with her work. That's the truth that my boss had asked me to deny: that a body, a human, an animal, can only take so much.

For writer Esmé Weijun Wang, that truth is hard to cover up. In "I'm Chronically Ill and Afraid of Being Lazy," an essay she wrote for *Elle*'s online magazine, Wang describes going from a caffeinated workaholic to someone who physically can't do as much as she'd like. She peppers the piece with photos. "Instead of bragging online and in person about how much work I've accomplished," she notes, "I post selfies from my bed, as if to prove that I am, indeed, ill."[6]

In her workaholic days, Wang used to pride herself on waking up at four in the morning to write for four hours before heading to the office. When things like limb pain and vomiting crept into her workday, she at first chalked it up to her coffee intake and her lack of computer ergonomics. After all, she writes, she was surrounded by "people who humblebragged about how little sleep they'd gotten the night before and used the phrases 'lean and scrappy' to describe not only our company culture, but themselves." When the symptoms became more worrisome—pain, fainting, trouble walking in a straight line—she finally went through medical testing. A doctor diagnosed her with late-stage Lyme disease, and she began various forms of treatment.

"This," she writes, "is where I am now: too sick to go back to full-time work, freelancing and building a small online business with what energy I do have, and still alive enough to know how much I'm not doing."

Wang seems acutely aware of the gulf between what she would like to do and what in reality her body can accomplish:

> I can, on most days, work for approximately two or three hours, using bits of time here and there with breaks for rest. I can't, on most days, function well after approximately 2 p.m., which is when I begin to develop fevers, moderate to severe nausea, weakness, fatigue, and a cornucopia of other symptoms that I never get used to, no matter how often they come to call.

Even while dealing with these extreme medical symptoms on a regular basis, Wang wants to do more. "After all, my work ethic and ambition haven't gone anywhere," she writes. That she is doing less than what she used to, or perhaps less than what others seem to be doing, feels to her like laziness—or "like a moral failing."

I can relate to Wang. On days when my own Lyme disease acts up, my joints suddenly sore, or when I have to trudge an hour to the hospital for my twice-yearly cancer checkup or am inexplicably exhausted despite needing to get work done, I feel as though I've done something wrong. And I wonder if a better person than I could just power through it. Am I just being lazy, deep down?

This, it turns out, is what Wang asks herself, too. "My deep fear," she writes, "is that I'm secretly slothful and am using chronic illness to disguise the sick rot of laziness within myself. Surely I can rouse myself from this bed and bring myself to my desk?"

The answer, clearly, is no, she can't. But like other young people who want that energetic go-getter vibe to be theirs again, who want to do what their peers are doing, Wang keeps asking herself to try harder, to try to negate the possibility that her health is limiting her career. To look up at that glass ceiling and try to wipe away the fog.

For some young women I've met, their current job works all right with their health needs, but a switch to a new career would probably be untenable. April, the twenty-eight-year-old with many surgical scars, has worked as a tenant organizer and a street-vendor organizer in New York City. Shortly after having surgery to get a pacemaker, she pushed herself, posting flyers around buildings and holding meetings with tenants. In hindsight, she says, "I probably shouldn't have done that much." Aside from the pressure she puts on herself, her current position is flexible enough that she can go into work late when she has appointments. "With both my jobs, I had a lot of control over my schedule," she says. But, she adds, "There's a part of me that could never be—there's a part of me that wants to be a teacher, but there's a part of me that's like, I could never. As a teacher, you have to be there at a certain time," and there isn't that flexibility, she says. "It does make me nervous for a different type of job." Despite her desire to try teaching, she says, "the idea is scary to me to have such a regimented work schedule."

Teaching is also what Tina used to do. Tina, who lives in a small town in the middle of the country, has both endometriosis and PCOS, or polycystic ovary syndrome. She's usually a vivacious, out-and-about, working-hard-and-getting-things-done type, but is now struck by debilitating pain and fatigue. She taught special ed for five years, then left when she started to burn out—not from the students, she says, but from the lack of administrative support. Now she's working at a small company run by a friend of her boyfriend's. And in addition to the chronic health conditions that wear her down, she's also about to have a baby.

"Work is part of your identity," she says, "but with the fatigue of being a mom and a chronic illness, I don't know what that's going to look like." One thing Tina does know is that she wants to work. She wants a career. She could stay at home, but she doesn't want to. On the other hand, she knows that her two conditions, combined with the new baby, might put some careers out of reach.

Back when she was teaching, she says, "I would be so fatigued, I would get home and put the peanut butter in the freezer. I had like five brain cells left. I couldn't string a sentence together. I don't want to be like *that* again."

Where is the line, I always wonder, between attending to one's health and maintaining or starting a career? Tina thinks of career as tied to her identity. So does Esmé Weijun Wang, and so do I. There's the ideal, and then there's the reality of what we can do without completely ravaging our health.

I visit the office of Tracey Revenson, a professor of psychology and area head of health psychology and clinical science at Hunter College and the Graduate Center at the City University of New York. She tells me that one of her doctoral students is looking at financial stress in young adults with serious health conditions. Revenson confirms that the stress is not just about the money, but is tied to identity, to growing up. When younger adults are hit with things like cancer before they've even begun their career, they think, Will I be able to have a satisfying career and support myself?

In some cases, young women weigh the risks and decide that their career can indeed come first. A woman I met in the United States got an incredible job offer for a project in China. But she has ulcerative colitis: her doctor said no. He reminded her that she needed checkups with him every three months and that she needed her prescriptions. She just couldn't live so far away, he said.

She considered it. Her colitis affects her everyday life, she knew, but she also didn't want to give up on this huge opportunity. She decided that despite her doctor's warning, it was important for her career to go. She would have her boyfriend mail the prescriptions to her in China, and she would come home as often as possible. She went to China and made it work, but had she listened to her physician, that whole new part of her career would have been off-limits because of her health.

––––

Sophie is an early-career scientist and the type of conversationalist for whom the term *bubbly* was invented. She was also born with HIV.

"My life expectancy was age two," she says. "So, going on twenty-seven, that was fun to prove doctors wrong."

Sophie got into a National Institutes of Health (NIH) medical trial right before her second birthday. Every birthday, she thanks her mother for enrolling her in it. Otherwise, she says, "God knows what would have happened to me." She sounds a bit in awe of the decisions that adults made for her when she was a toddler: that her biological mother, a drug user, had put her up for adoption and that her adoptive parents had fostered many children but for some reason chose to fully adopt her. She is also grateful that her birth mother, whom she's still in touch with, at first wouldn't give permission to let Sophie move away, but finally did, and for the whole series of events that led her to the NIH trial that probably saved her life.

Her career choice, she says, is informed by her experience as a kid. For years, she went to NIH frequently: at first every other month, then every three months, then every six. She was doing so well by second or third grade that she could finally stop going. But then, two years later, she got pancreatitis for a second time. By then, she had to return to NIH. By this point in elementary school, she knew what CD4 cells, or T-cells, were. She knew lots of facts about bodies, immune systems, and viruses—things the other kids her age didn't know.

Going through HIV-related sicknesses and treatments as a child, she thought she wanted to be a doctor.

In college, she had trouble finding the right internship to help her become a physician. So her doctor at NIH invited her to be an intern there. There was one major caveat: it would be all bench work, meaning work in a lab. She would work on the research side of medicine, not the side engaged with patients. Sophie thought she was too much of a people person. No way would she enjoy working in a lab setting. But it turned out that she loved doing biomedical research. She found it satisfying to get results in the lab—results that would later help doctors and their patients.

As for the outgoingness that she'd hoped to use with patients as a physician, she says, "I bring my spunky personality everywhere I go." And so she did two internships in the lab, chatting away with her colleagues, and studying, as she puts it, "the monkey version of HIV" to help researchers understand the human virus. There, among the glass tubes and instruments, she began to really understand what was going on in her own body. While she had initially planned on studying to be a pediatrician, she knew that whether as a doctor or a scientist, she wanted to focus on infectious disease.

For a while, she still held on to the idea of being a physician, until she realized that she was good at the science side and that she could bring something unusual to it. There's a disconnect between medical doctors, society, and researchers, she tells me. As someone with HIV, she understands the patient side of infectious disease in a way that many of her colleagues do not.

For her master's degree, Sophie studied gonorrhea. When we met, she was just starting her PhD program and was at the moment studying HIV—the human version of the disease. It's an adventure, she says, to be working on her own virus.

But fascinating and strange as it feels to be studying what's in her own body, it's complicated to be who she is in a biomedical research setting.

"I'm a young black female working in a predominately white and Asian and Indian field," she says.

"And male, right?" I ask.

"Oh, especially male, oh my gosh. I am the minority on any level."

"I'm very . . . what you would call . . . I'm very pro-black," Sophie tells me. "I try not to throw that out there too much." But she has seen how her own identity as a black woman comes up at work, especially after a string of police shootings and the rise of the Black Lives Matter movement. On top of navigating working in a nonblack space amid racial injustice ("My biological mother calls me her little Black Panther," she says), she has to navigate colleagues who don't truly understand her disease. She's heard HIV researchers talk about patients in a way that makes it painfully obvious that they have no idea what it's like.

"So envision me and my black-power-ness, and being awakened, especially this year," she says, referring to Black Lives Matter, ". . . but at the same time still having to deal with people's ignorance about HIV."

And what about disclosing her health status to those at work or in her doctoral program?

"I don't actually know who knows," she says, "because I wrote about it in my essay." In her grad school applications, she wrote about what drove her to study infectious disease. Later, when she told a teacher in her master's program that she was positive, he said he already knew.

Now, in her PhD program, she wonders who else might know. She wonders, too, if people make assumptions or if they don't believe that she was born with it. Over the years, Sophie has noticed the difference in people's reactions when they find out that she was born with HIV and didn't contract it later, as if somehow she were absolved from the blame that these same people would heap on those who got it at a later age. Just because her colleagues study disease, she's found, doesn't mean they're exempt from this type of thinking.

There's also her fear that people she doesn't want to know about her health will find out. When she goes to the infectious disease clinic on campus, for her own health care, she doesn't want her peers to see her. And yet, on one of the days we speak, Sophie has just run into someone. The student asked her, "What are you doing around here?"

But even though she'd known that person for a year, she didn't necessarily want to explain. When she's working in the lab, that brings a whole set of fears, too.

"I get sick often. I get headaches often," she says, and she wonders, "What if I get sick in the lab?" At one point, she got thrush, a fungal infection, in her throat, from not taking her medicine regularly enough. She was terrified. She knew that people couldn't see inside her throat, but if she got sicker and she was at work, colleagues would likely start to ask what was wrong.

"I just don't want to be treated differently," she says. She doesn't particularly like that people who do know about her health are extra delicate with her.

Her advisors are trying to be better mentors, she says. They also always ask how her health is at the moment. She seems glad that they care, but disappointed that they have tunnel vision. When they're trying to check in about how her personal life is going, their questions are always about her HIV.

When it comes to supervisors who know her health status, she says, "It's wonderful that they're understanding, but I wonder how many times they think I might get sick. I don't want to be that person who always uses it as an excuse."

———

"I'm going to sound corny," Brenda warns me when I ask for her thoughts on being a young woman in a high-powered career in Washington, both before and after her rare neurological disease began.

"I wanted to break through the barriers," she says. "I wanted to dedicate myself to paving a path for the next generation of Latinas. I was walking along the path that other Latina women had laid for me. And, I was doing it well. I knew I was fighting harder than most others had to fight for the same things. But, I was—and still am— willing to push harder than the day before to make it. And then the disease came."

Now, "I find myself overcompensating for my disease. I work longer hours than my colleagues," she says—or, technically, types. Because her disease can affect her speech, we're accommodating it by using G-chat instead of speaking out loud. "I am willing to do tasks normally assigned to junior associates, because I want to prove my worth. I want to not only do my job, but I want to go above and beyond to show that despite all of my special needs, I'm worth it."

Brenda's symptoms started when she held a high-powered role: press secretary for the Joint Economic Committee of the US Congress. When we meet, she's at a DC firm that works on coalition building, lobbying, and strategic communications in pursuit of progressive public policy. At thirty-three, Brenda is the director. I hope she doesn't mind the term, I tell her, but I say "high-powered" because she's clearly done a lot of badass things at a young age.

"It seems there's the regular glass ceiling," I say to her, "then the additional one when you get sick. Then there's yet another if you're a woman of color. And the list goes on." But, I ask, since she's a fellow word person, someone who's crafted communications for senators, does a more accurate metaphor come to mind?

"I don't think that the glass ceiling is totally accurate," she says. "At least you can see through the glass ceiling." Instead, she says, "I'm a woman, and I see a glass ceiling that I need to break through. I'm a Latina, and I see a wall that I have to figure out how to get over or find the one small door somewhere. I am disabled, and I now have an obstacle course before me that I have to navigate. And now I have a speech impediment, and I have to figure out how to sing an opera."

Despite all this, she feels lucky.

"I am a female, Hispanic, disabled Jew," she says. But, she adds, "my workplace celebrates diversity and has gone above and beyond."

That doesn't stop her, though, from putting in extra time, taking on extra tasks, and trying to prove, over and over, that she deserves to be where she is.

———

Eileen was already working at a hospital when she found a lump in her breast. She was thirty-four and raising three young daughters. At the university medical center where she oversaw human resources and academic affairs for the cardiology department, she walked over to the mammography area to get the lump examined.

"You're too young," the person at the front desk told her. "Another six years." But Eileen had a lump, even though she was under forty. Once she finally persuaded the receptionist that she needed to be seen and had a mammogram, she could tell from the looks on people's faces that something was up. They immediately called in a sonogram technician. Eileen, it turns out, had stage 2 triple-negative breast cancer: a particularly dangerous strain that disproportionately affects younger, premenopausal women, as well as those of African American or Latinx descent.

This subtype of the disease, as the Triple Negative Breast Cancer Foundation explains, can be particularly aggressive. In other subtypes, estrogen receptors, progesterone receptors, and human epidermal growth factor 2 receptors fuel the disease, meaning doctors can target them for successful treatment. But in patients like Eileen, the tumor is negative for those three receptors, and treatments that target them don't help much.

"I'm a Latina of African descent from the Dominican Republic," she says, "and I was thirty-four"—a prime target for the disease in terms of both heritage and age. She had a lumpectomy to remove the tumor. But then, just a few weeks later, during Breast Cancer Awareness Month, she happened to see something about a woman who had the cancer come back in her other breast. That woman was also in her thirties. So Eileen called her surgeon again—a doctor who, she adds, now also happens to be her boss. But we'll get to that in a moment.

She asked for a bilateral mastectomy. After the surgeon had removed her breasts, Eileen started on five and a half months of chemotherapy. She took a ten-month disability leave from her job. But she still went to the hospital frequently, now as a patient. There, she'd see acquaintances from work in the halls, "and they would just look down," she says, "or they would try not to look me in the eyes."

But wait, I ask. These are her own colleagues, people who work in a hospital every day, and they can't handle it? Aren't these the very people who work to make sick people feel better? Meanwhile, Eileen, weak from treatment, is now carrying the extra weight of worrying about her colleagues. "Oh my god, I hope I don't run into anyone," she remembers thinking, "because I don't want to make *them* feel uncomfortable."

"I think that's a very woman thing," I say.

"Yeah, that's for sure! I would walk in with my husband, and I would say, 'Oh my god, they're not going to know what to say.'" Her husband's reply: "Why do you care about that?"

Indeed, one of her colleagues confirmed all this out loud in the hall. "She said, 'I don't know what to say,'" Eileen remembers, "and she just dashed away!"

"This was a very physical disease," Eileen says. "I had no hair, no eyebrows. I lost in the process forty pounds. . . . I'm not a psychotherapist or anything, but I'm thinking when you're in your thirties, nobody wants to think about that." She figures that she was a reminder of mortality for her colleagues—even colleagues who were used to being around people with illnesses.

I tell her about the essay I read in the *Washington Post*, the one in which Katherine Russell Rich's editor tells her she reminds the whole office of mortality and that this is why no one wants to work with her. Eileen says she relates. At the same time, she has an empathetic and generous outlook on the colleagues who scurried away at the sight of her.

"I certainly don't want to think about dying when I have little children," she admits. Still, the way her coworkers acted around her sounds almost comically unprofessional. After her treatment and a clinical trial, Eileen developed a blood clot that became more serious than the cancer itself. The clot could have "detonated" in an instant, and she had to give herself daily injections to treat it. With this other serious health concern, it was the same story again. The doctor treating her for the clot, she says, "would just sort of make the mad dash when I walked [down the hall], and he was my caregiving doctor."

About her colleagues who ran away from her, she says, "clearly the answer is yes, you should have compassion, you should have that level of professionalism where you should know how to interact." But she remembers what she learned from a pediatrician with a sick daughter: doctors can't care for their own loved ones. Too much emotion. And so, she says, "the only answer that I can give you is that maybe that is the case," that the situation was too close for comfort.

Despite all this, she felt lucky—a word that keeps coming up with the women I meet. She had been working there for eight or nine years already, had established herself professionally, and enjoyed a close bond with her own staff members. They were the ones who, as she puts it, picked her up off the ground. Even when she was in the infusion room getting chemotherapy, her staff would show up and ask for her advice on a work issue. They knew how important her job was to her, and they kept her in the loop while she was on leave trying to get rid of the cancer. And it was in the infusion room that her career began to shift in unexpected ways.

During her own treatment, Eileen educated herself on nutrition: the benefits of vegetables, the health risks of too much sugar.

"It was almost by mistake," she says of how her illness changed her career. "I would be in the chemotherapy suite, and I would see women eating cake and even the food they would give you in there." It wasn't healthy, she says. She wanted to advocate for patients and help them learn they had agency in what they did with their bodies. And there was more she started to notice.

"The hospital is in Washington Heights, which is largely an immigrant community," she says, yet the doctors don't know the language. "I was just getting pulled into conversations." By speaking Spanish and English, and helping the physicians and patients understand each other, she says, "I was just a patient and an advocate at the same time."

"Health care is not designed for the poor. It's not designed for women of color. It's not designed for the undocumented," she says. And, she was seeing, it wasn't designed for younger women, either.

"I walked into a support group . . . and I walked right out," she remembers. "Everyone was older than me. It was a terrible experience."

Not only was Eileen the only one her age, but the meeting was held in a basement. She and other patients undergoing chemo were already vomiting constantly from the treatment, and here the support group was, next to the smell of hot basement garbage. Many of the women, who were all much older than she was, were crying. Very somber. So Eileen immediately left.

As a patient and an observer, Eileen was starting to see "the horrors" within the health-care system. No one was doing outreach to younger women, many of whom had her triple-negative subtype. And although she was the target demographic for this type of breast cancer, the photos in the literature looked nothing like her: all the women pictured were white.

She also saw that a lot of the women with breast cancer were immigrants with very low socioeconomic status. That's what really made her want to be an advocate in a more official capacity. She found herself having to remind her coworkers that these patients, many of whom worked as cleaning women, had rights just like anybody else, regardless of their income level.

And she realized she could help even more. She worked on becoming more public about her own story and her advocacy. The university was holding a conference for women of color with cancer and asked her to be a speaker. Her surgeon, whose own sister had died of breast cancer at thirty-seven, saw how strong an advocate Eileen had become. He said he wanted her to work in his department because nobody else had the passion she had for patients' rights.

"I said, 'No, it has to be the right role,'" Eileen recalls. "'I'm an HR manager. Let's get the role right.'" It took a year, but she and her surgeon—the one who's now her boss—worked out a job description and went through the necessary steps, and Eileen became an official patient navigator.

I ask if she's the first one to have this role at this well-established university hospital. In name only, she says, did the role previously exist. The previous navigator didn't do what she's doing now. Eileen creates inclusive workshops for cancer patients from many demographics. She brings in experts to teach patients how to make healthy and tasty meals, and she makes sure that young women don't feel as out of place as she did. She also ensures that the resources are available in Spanish. She's the first patient navigator to do all that.

"Patient navigation is sort of this new thing that's emerging from a health-care system that's spread too thin," she says. "There's not enough resources." The so-called patient navigator who was at the hospital when Eileen was diagnosed in 2008 didn't get to fulfill the title. In a place that was understaffed, the navigator ended up as an extra person at the front desk to help check patients in or tell them when to get undressed.

"She was basically like an office clerk or a medical assistant, a secretary," Eileen says. Now, when people ask Eileen to make an appointment for a patient or do something else outside her role, she sets boundaries. She doesn't want to become just like the navigator before her, who never had a moment to actually help patients through their illness.

There's another type of navigator, too, Eileen says, a volunteer who "waits for a crying lady, offers her chocolate, tea, or coffee. But it's usually an older white lady who has nothing else to do," she says, "and is probably married to a rich guy."

While her assumptions about the volunteers' relationships may not be accurate, she makes a point. A young immigrant woman who lives in New York City's Washington Heights neighborhood, Eileen says, or a young woman of color probably won't relate to this much older white person at all when she is upset, even if the volunteer is well-meaning. Eileen remembers encountering such a woman after her own doctor's visit. The chasm between them was large. (At the same time, though, outside the hospital, she says, she related to older women more than she related to some of her friends.)

Now that Eileen is on the staff side again, she puts together workshops and environments that feel inviting to young women like her. Instead of a support group in the putrid-smelling basement, where no one is young and everyone is in tears, she has a group in which the word *cancer* seldom even comes up and where the mood is light and helpful, not somber.

"We have an Alvin Ailey dancer come in, and who's crying then?" she says. "Or we have a chef come in teaching vegetable-based cooking. Who's crying?" When women have questions about reconstructive surgery, she even lets them touch her implants to see what they feel like.

Her own diagnosis, she says, made her and her husband realize they weren't going to live forever. Both of them shifted their priorities and their focus at work after her cancer.

"I think all of this came out of being young and still having the time to make a career change," she says.

And now in her position, she, too, sees women from her workplace suddenly showing up as patients, just as she once did. But, she says, she runs toward these women, not away from them.

———

I meet with Victoria Rodriguez-Roldan, who at twenty-eight is director of the transgender and gender-nonconforming justice project at the National LGBTQ Task Force. When we meet for sushi, Rodriguez-

Roldan is working on several social justice issues within the trans and gender-nonconforming world, with an emphasis on the intersection between trans rights and disability justice, including labor and employment discrimination.

"I feel like it says a lot about how we treat mental health disabilities in our society," she says, " . . . that I was out and very much open about my being trans, very, very early on in college, but I honestly didn't quite—didn't open up about anything on my mental health outside of perhaps a very select group of people." Rodriguez-Roldan didn't reveal that she had bipolar disorder until shortly after she finished law school. She was, at the time, "more scared of the consequences of *that* coming out, so to speak." As a law student, she suspected that to pass the bar, it would be easier if nobody knew about her mental health disabilities. The bar, she says, can make you disclose hospital records—and significant discrimination and stigmatization exists around mental health in the legal profession. While being trans is often stigmatized and discriminated against, she worried more about people's reactions to her bipolar disorder.

These days, Rodriguez-Roldan, who also has developed some physical health issues since then, gets a certain thrill from outing herself in professional settings. As a director at a national organization based in DC, she regularly interacts with members of Congress and other high-ranking officials. Sometimes, she says, a powerful person on Capitol Hill will mention bipolar and other mental health disabilities to Rodriguez-Roldan in a *those*-people-with-mental-illness kind of way. "You mean people like me?" she'll reply, deadpan. The brief uncomfortable silence that follows, she tells me, can be priceless. She gets to watch a powerful decision maker reconfigure their concept of mental health and perhaps shift, ever so slightly, the idea of "us" versus "them."

"Sometimes I feel like I can't do certain things and I avoid them when I don't feel safe," writes Emily, a young woman who identifies as Chinese and lives in San Francisco. She has multiple sclerosis.

"I'm a filmmaker, so it's definitely not a desk job," she tells me. "When I'm out in the field, I'm always on my feet and I have to be careful that I don't suddenly let my legs give out, especially when I'm near expensive equipment. It's a constant battle to remember to be aware of my surroundings."

She also remembers an internship at which she was learning to do tech on a stage. "I had to just let my boss know that I didn't feel safe being on a three-foot platform with no railings," she says. "After I 'came out' about having MS, he was actually a bit upset with me that I didn't tell him sooner. I was glad he understood, but it also meant that I wasn't able to learn how to use the cameras and stage equipment."

I ask what it's like to work in a field known as a white boys' club. "Being a woman of color has never been an issue for me," she says. "I myself don't even register how few Asian filmmakers there are when I'm working. If anything, I feel more alone as a woman on set than as an Asian. Film sets are fairly diverse in San Francisco, but there aren't usually many females around." And, she says, "for the most part my coworkers don't even remember that I have MS, so they treat me like how they would anyone. But sometimes I'm asked to do things and I have to remind them that I can't. We're all pretty friendly at work, but I do often feel judged, as if my illness is not being taken seriously or they think I'm just using MS as an excuse."

And so, she says, "I try to keep it to myself. For the most part, I try my best to be 'normal' unless I don't feel safe. But sometimes I do push myself a little too far because I don't want to be deemed useless."

Another woman I interviewed, a thirty-year-old named Jayde, doesn't want to be deemed useless, either. Jayde has familial adenomatous polyposis, a disease that causes polyps as well as cancer in many parts of the body and which has upended many of her organs and years of her life. Money is tight, too. She tried to raise some through a crowdfunding site to help pay for her trips to specialists in other parts of the country, but she didn't raise much, and she can't afford as many visits as she probably needs. She's had her colon removed and countless other procedures, and when we meet, she admits that she's been putting off brain surgery. It's just been too much. I ask if her health has affected jobs for her or taken away a dream career.

"I tried to live my dream multiple times," she says. "My main goal as a child was to follow my grandfather's [footsteps]. He was in the air force. I'm afraid of airplanes . . . but I did want to become a JAG [Judge Advocate General's Corps] officer, and get into law, and make it to the White House. Not to be the president of the United States, of course, but I saw myself doing [big] things in the air force and everything. I wanted that uniform so bad." So very bad, she tells me, that she made an attempt despite knowing the reality: that her body was against her.

"I tried—I actually tried to lie my way through it," she says. She marvels at her own tenacity: "I tried to still get them to come out to my house and do an interview. And my stupid self, I'm like, 'They're not gonna look that much into my medical history. It's only the *government*—they don't have your information!'" She laughs for a moment at how far she went to convince herself that the authorities would magically not discover her health issues.

When the air force turned her down because of her disease, she tried to convince them again. "But you don't understand, I'm strong willed, even if I'm sick," she remembers saying to them. "I'm stronger than you think I am." But she didn't make it past the health requirements.

After her dream of being a JAG officer was extinguished, she enrolled in a local community college. She loved her first semester. It opened her eyes to history and art, she says. She felt herself growing as a person. But her disease was still there. She had to trick her body by taking her medicine without eating food, since food after colon surgery tended to disrupt her day. After her second semester of trying to balance her body and her desire to learn, she had to drop out.

"I said, 'Okay, let me try to just go out and get a job,'" she says. She applied to numerous places and started working at a clothing store while also doing shifts at Applebee's. The clothing store was great, she says. The owners were wonderful and generously gave their employees wardrobes. They sent her to fancy business dinners and made the job exciting. And one of Jayde's bosses, it so happened, had ulcers, meaning he had to eat on a similarly restrictive diet and schedule as Jayde did. Having a supervisor with similar restrictions, even for a less extreme condition, helped her work around her health with a little more ease. Still, she was pushing her insides toward an unsustainable rhythm. The job was great, but the schedule was untenable.

"I was able to trick my body for a good year," she says. "And then it caught up with me." Jayde still wanted an education past high school, though, so she tried school again, this time from home.

"I did DeVry," she says, referring to the university's online program. "It's just as expensive as a regular two-year college. Had to get loans and all that stuff. Extremely expensive." She also lost her health insurance and had to start paying out of pocket for her medical expenses. But she couldn't afford to do that and pay back her student loans. When the school said she couldn't attend classes unless she paid back one of her loans, that was it. She had to keep up with her doctors' appointments, and so the medical costs won out over school. Then, she says, even though she wishes she were working or taking classes again, she had to apply for disability. "I need income," she says.

But, she adds, "I'm not one of those people that actually wants to collect disability and be lazy." And there it is again: that fear of laziness, even though Jayde has, without question, tried to work in various fields and pushed herself, hard. As she's talking, I think about how Jayde, a young black woman, might have fewer stereotypes thrown at her if she were white. How, instead, our society makes assumptions about her that she now worries about.

Jayde's disease is rare. But her lack of money, despite her best efforts, isn't. She is one of countless Americans who work hard to get an education and start a career but who are derailed in part by health-care costs. On the surface, her disease may seem to be the obstacle. But the more I heard about her experience, the more it became clear that racial and structural inequality and our country's unaffordable health-care and education systems have played a huge role. Had Jayde been able to pay back her loans and keep going to school from home—had she come from a higher-income background or lived in a country where college is low cost or free—things may have been very different. She might have secured a job that accommodated her health and let her work from home when she needed. Instead, she's forced to eke by, even though what she wants is a career.

———

For Jayde, passing off her health situation as nothing too out of the ordinary seemed a bit easier when her boss had one, too. At least, up to a point. Other young women make similar calculations: how much they think they can divulge without weirding people out at work—or, worse, losing their job.

A friend leads me to a blog by Samantha Kittle, a young actress and writer who had also had a brain tumor and was now posting about her ongoing experience.[7] In one entry, she connects her career and her appearance. In the photos on her blog, Kittle looks healthy after her surgery; there would be no way to tell what she has been through. That is, unless the scar that plows through her hair is showing. She describes the changes to her appearance after surgery:

> My hair will always be kept short. I will never be able to grow it and have *my own* long hair. No more ponytails (made of my real hair). No more hairstyles (of my hair). It's wigs and scarves and hats and headbands from now on.
>
> It's not a vanity thing, but a practical thing. My current short hair cut, when left to its own devices may be manageable with lots of effort, but no more bad hair days that I can throw my hair up into a ponytail or bun. It can be covered, that's it. When met with minimal effort my short hair cut, at best, appears unkempt and reveals bald spots/scars that I am not ashamed of. Professionally, however, it is not a permanent option. I cannot simply brush it and move on. . . .
>
> Again, it's also not just vanity or the age-old bullshit about how much pressure is put on women's appearance. I understand that in my current line of work as a low-level medical assistant for a large nonprofit health organization that I should not be at work with crazy hair. It makes me look unprofessional and unkempt. It reflects poorly on my office.

And, Kittle admits, as a patient herself, she too would be unsettled by a nurse or physician's assistant whose hair looked like hers now does. So she covers it up and conforms.

———

Some women, though, feel they must be open about their experiences at work—even their baldness (albeit temporary). And some of them get positive feedback from their peers.

When I meet Miriam, her voice immediately strikes me as warm and real. The El Paso high school where she's the new assistant principal has just let out for the day, and she's raced to our phone call as quickly as she could. She used to be a teacher before she was promoted, and the new, somewhat daunting position seems to mean a lot to her. The school community means a great deal to her, too, especially after she had to tell her students that she had cancer.

Miriam had been trying to get doctors to pay attention to her strange symptoms for fifteen months, but she kept being told she was fine. Finally, a few weeks before her thirtieth birthday, she learned she had stage 3 breast cancer. She was stuck not only with what she feared was a death sentence but also with the burden of explaining to her class what was happening. The school year was ending when she received the news, and when she returned from her treatment to meet her new class, she was bald. She walked into school the first day with a scarf on her head, explained that she had cancer, then came in the next day with her head visibly bare.

Many of the students to whom she had revealed her health status cried with her. Some of them had a parent, grandparent, or sibling with cancer, she says, but the students had never been able to ask questions. Whereas it had been a taboo subject in their families, Miriam, their teacher, was providing a safe place for them to ask about something scary.

And many fellow teachers and staff members approached her as well. They confided that they, too, had cancer, but had wanted to keep it a secret at work. She was stunned to realize how many colleagues had been hiding the same illness. Even parents of her students started coming in and telling her about a lump they had. Although Miriam couldn't believe they hadn't told anyone else, she was glad to help.

She decided to be open with everyone at the school, thinking that the more people talk about taboo illnesses, the more hope there is in finding a remedy or at least support.

"A lot of fear comes from not knowing," she says. She describes an interview she did with *Latino Leaders*. The magazine featured Miriam in a story about a partnership between the publication and the cancer center where Miriam had been treated. There, she's photographed alongside an oncologist and a surgeon, discussing efforts to engage the Latinx community in cancer awareness. Miriam wants to help her community learn ways to prevent cancer through lifestyle choices, as well as help demystify what it's like to go through the disease and its treatment. As she talks to me about promoting awareness, it's apparent that much of her effort has been while she's at work. She allowed her students, their families, and her colleagues to see her at her lowest point, she says, and by being transparent and open at her job, she believes that she has helped spread knowledge about the disease.

Miriam isn't the only woman who feels strongly about disclosing health issues at work. Vita, the young woman with multiple sclerosis whose date pushed her away, tells me that the MS Society suggests keeping one's health status a secret when it comes to jobs. Even though there are some legal protections against discrimination, she says, it's really difficult to prove. But Vita makes a point to talk about her MS at work. She doesn't want to hide it, and in any case, she says, she has to go to the doctor often, so people would notice. Vita works in the nonprofit world. If a workplace discriminates against people because of a disability, she says, she's not interested in working there. She has had coworkers ask in hushed tones if she's okay when she comes back from a doctor's appointment. Sometimes it's an appointment related to MS, but other times it's a regular old dental cleaning. People forget, she says, that just because she has extra doctors to go to for MS doesn't mean she's immune to going to the dentist.

Sometimes, though, it doesn't matter whether a young woman wants to hide her health issues or keep them private at work. If an issue is visible, it can feel like the power has shifted.

———

"Isn't that right, Gimpy?" my supervisor said. I thought I'd misheard. I had not.

After romanticizing, for years, what being a temporary US Census worker would show me—my neighborhood, my country, humanity with a capital *H*—I stood in the basement of a public library with a group of other trainees. I had just undergone joint surgery a few weeks before and was still in pain but, for the job interview, had decided to leave my crutches at home. The surgeon let me walk a tiny bit without them, and since I thought I was vying for a door-to-door gig, I'd thought, *Who would hire me like this?*

So I paid for a taxi. At twenty-six, I usually opted for the much more affordable subway, but then I would need the crutches, and I didn't want to seem less-than. Even though the job was a federal one—even though there are laws to protect people from discrimination in hiring—I wasn't sure if my surgery and temporary crutches would count under the Americans with Disabilities Act or any other protective policy. The problem was, the interview was in a part of Lower Manhattan that the cab driver didn't know how to navigate, an area of the financial district where the streets get narrow and, instead of numbers, have names. He drove around a bit, seemed frustrated, then said, "I don't know where that street is, miss. I can't find it. Gonna just let you out here."

Without my crutches, I looked like a completely healthy, mobile young woman. But for all I knew, he was letting me out ten blocks away, a distance I wasn't supposed to walk without crutches for another few weeks. "Uh, the thing is, I actually just had surgery," I said. "So . . . I can't really walk. That's why I took a cab." I braced for the usual you-look-young-to-me response. The guy, I think, was confused. "I didn't bring my crutches," I said. "I need to get as close to that street as possible, if we can, because otherwise I can't really get there."

I felt bad. Neither of us, at the time, had a way to look at a map. I had a flip phone and a scribbled-down cross street and address. The cab driver, who I'd thought might not mind driving around more with the meter racking up dollars, seemed instead annoyed. "I don't know where Gold Street is from here!" he shouted. I don't know why he shouted. We were in an area where the city gets a little less gridlike and predictable, but I had hoped the cab driver would know the street. My eyes felt hot. I asked him again, explained again that I couldn't walk there, even if someone could point me in the right direction. But he didn't want to drive anymore, even though the fare would have increased in his favor. I didn't know what to do. I paid him and got out. I asked someone on the street for directions. I walked. At first, I felt okay.

Two blocks later, I felt my hip ache. Three blocks later, I was experiencing searing pain. By the time I got to the census headquarters, I knew I might have done damage to the still-healing incision that went all the way from the top layer of my skin to the inside of my hip bone. There was nothing to do but pretend I was fine, or so I thought. My goal while healing from surgery was this: act like I was a sprightly young thing, and make sure nobody thought I had health issues.

In the end, the person who hired me said that I had tested out of knocking door-to-door, the job I actually wanted. I had scored high enough that I would instead be managing a group of fifteen to twenty people who would do the actual apartment visits. After getting the job, I showed up on my first day on foot yet again, no visible sign of my surgery, and met my new supervisor and coworkers at our training session. Then, after a great deal of pain, I learned from my physical therapist that, not surprisingly, I had to use the crutches again. I'd gotten off them far too soon. The next day, I self-consciously crutched into the room where my boss was continuing to train us, and, bam, I heard the slur. "Isn't that right, Gimpy?" he said, looking around to see if he'd made any of my coworkers laugh.

And again, a minute later, as we took turns reading something out loud: "Paragraph two, Gimpy." I felt fiery, but said nothing.

I could have told my supervisor, a wise guy who thought he was magnificently intelligent and certainly more worldly than he really was, that what he had said was illegal. I could have said, "Wait, what?"—that gentler kind of calling someone out. But I just sat there, next to my crutches, and made a face that suggested I was only casually annoyed by a comment that was actually offensive, not to mention childish and mean. Or maybe, more likely, I just looked scared.

Some of the other people in the training seemed to perk up a bit at the comment. At some point, I think, one of them said something on my behalf. "Oh come on," my supervisor said, "I wouldn't have said that to you if it was permanent." In other words, chill out.

He kept it up until, perhaps, he noticed that nobody laughed.

Whether or not it was permanent, I wanted to tell him, he shouldn't have said it at a work meeting. Or at all. Probably ever. It seemed even stranger that this was at a federal job meant to take a census of all the people in the country. *Everybody Counts!* the slogan went. But I said nothing. It's hard to get your words out when your boss says something that smarts in front of all your colleagues, even if you suspect that your colleagues are on your side. This man seemed to feel some license as my supervisor, license that perhaps came from my being a young, healthy-looking woman in my twenties—this idea that my condition wasn't permanent and that, therefore, a slur was okay.

I didn't want to feel embarrassed, because I had done nothing embarrassing. But the word *gimpy* hovered around me like a swarm of bees I couldn't shake, following me the next few days at work.

Those who have a visible disability while trying to find work or keep their job have to navigate a system that wasn't built for them. They have colleagues and supervisors who may not understand or care to understand their situation. And people with disabilities feel the pressure to work "just like anybody else" even when workplaces lack adequate accommodations—and even when people are hostile. Having an invisible health issue or disability comes with its own set of terrors. Do you reveal anything to your boss, or do you just hope nobody sees you as different, even if it means working extra hard and hiding a big part of yourself? Now that I'm a few years out from my last surgery, I still have pain every day. One thing that helps while I sit at a desk is a little foam wedge recommended to me by a biomechanics expert: something that goes on a regular chair to make the back of the seat higher. When I took the wedge with me to a conference for work, two things happened. My hip felt better, and I was in less overall pain—but also, I had to put a very visible weird contraption onto my chair every time I went to a session in a new room. I was there professionally, among people hungry to network, and I wondered whether people seeing me with an odd-looking device affected the chances of their networking with me.

Women in general make eighty cents for every dollar men do.[8] (Put another way, as the National Women's Law Center writes, "Based on today's wage gap, women would lose $418,800 over the course of a forty-year career" compared with men.)[9] When you're part of even more marginalized communities, the pay disparity is more shocking. Black women make about sixty-three cents on the dollar. Hispanic or Latinx women make fifty-four. Native Hawaiian women and Pacific Islanders make sixty cents, and American Indian and Alaska Native women make fifty-eight.[10] This differential is already egregious. Add in a cancer diagnosis, an autoimmune disease that drains your energy or changes how you can eat or move, major surgery, or bipolar disorder, and the odds become even more stacked against you.

Even for those of us who face relatively minor discrimination and structural inequality, being a young woman with a body that isn't doing the things people expect can jeopardize a job, a career, and a chance at a savings account. Just being a woman is enough. When you're discriminated against because of your background or skin color, too, finding equal opportunity becomes that much harder, financially and otherwise.

A few years ago, after always doing my taxes myself, I realized that my jobs and expenses were getting more complicated and that, as much as I didn't want to spend extra money, I needed a professional to help me. I met with someone who specializes in filing for writers, artists, and other freelancers who don't have traditional nine-to-fives. As we sat in his airy office space and went over the numbers I'd submitted, the tax preparer, a guy around my age, stopped.

"So, you wrote 'ten thousand dollars' under medical expenses," he said. "I'm guessing you accidentally typed a zero and you mean a thousand, right?"

But he was wrong. I had indeed spent ten thousand dollars in medical expenses: copays for physical therapists to ease joint problems and sports injuries, out-of-pocket payments to a Lyme disease specialist, and fees for other practitioners who helped me walk with less pain. That year had been unusually expensive for me, with health needs swallowing a larger percentage of my income than usual. But even if it surprised the tax preparer, who looked like someone I could just as easily have met at a party or a show, I was far from the only woman his age who had to devote that much to her health.

# PART 3

# It's Cool Guys
# I'm Totally Fine

In 2013, I was at physical therapy for some of my oh-so-lovely joint problems, icing my ankle after some exercises. Through the flimsy curtain separating patients, I heard a woman say she had been at a picnic the weekend before with friends. She realized that while everyone else was able to sit cross-legged with no problem for hours, she was unable to. Her hips and her knees hurt too much.

"I'm frustrated," I heard her tell the physical therapist. "I thought I wouldn't have to deal with that till I was in my seventies."

I listened closely. Related fully. But when she emerged from behind her side of the curtain, I saw that she was fifteen to twenty years older than I was.

I'm frustrated decades before you are, I wanted to say. I want to be the same fun person with my friends I've always been—the one who hangs out for hours at the picnic, laughs so hard that my drink comes out my nose. And sometimes I can't.

When you're young, you don't want to be the killjoy. If you're me, you want to feel free to do stupid, risky things like break into underground tunnels in Manhattan and, in near-darkness, dodge trains that speed toward you and don't know you're there. You want to walk on a bridge in western New York—a bridge that's only wide enough for the one-way train tracks it holds—knowing that your college crush and you will bond by casually risking your lives together, by flaunting just how death-proof you think you are. You get drawn toward being "just one of the guys," an expression you fundamentally disagree with as a feminist and yet use (and which for some reason keeps propelling you toward unsafe fun on active train tracks). You want to curl up with a book and read and sleep and eat, but you also want to feel a little dangerous on occasion, to meet strangers and travel to places your parents aren't happy about.

You want your danger to be a privilege, though: an adventure out in the world that you choose to take. Not something that comes from inside your own skin.

Walking down the street with Simon one night, I noticed I was avoiding the metal grating over the subway tunnel, gingerly stepping to the side so that my feet were on solid cement instead.

"Are you purposely avoiding stepping on the grates?" he asked. He'd noticed too. I had been trying to be slick about it, but it was obvious.

"Yeah," I said. "I realize that they're fine to walk on. But, you know, the city probably hasn't maintained them in forty years, and who knows, really." Then, sensing that this wasn't really the reason: "You know, when I was little, growing up in Manhattan, I used to stomp on the gratings, just jump all over them, stomping as if to tease the universe with my invincibility. Now, after all of the times I've had ridiculous medical stuff and almost died, I catch myself avoiding them."

I had grown into someone who knew I wasn't in control of whether I stayed alive from moment to moment. Whereas when I was younger I relished that testing, that teasing, of danger, my body now instinctively avoided it when it could, as if to compensate for all the times danger had struck and I'd had no choice.

In short, I now felt old.


"I'm 21 years old and I feel like I'm 50. I'm 50, I feel like I'm 90. I am only 22 and I feel like I am like 60 or 70 years old." These are some of the message-board comments Amy Berkowitz has collaged in *Tender Points*, a slim volume that explores Berkowitz's own fibromyalgia, the alienating nature of pain, and the possible connections between autoimmune disease and sexual assault.[1] The passage echoes the sentiments of many young women I've met, women who feel ancient compared with their healthier friends, who feel eighty even though they're thirty. Who feel off time, out of chronological step with their peers. As one researcher puts it in "Chronic Illness as Biographical Disruption," a frequently cited paper from the 1980s, being sick "involves a recognition of the worlds of pain and suffering, possibly even of death, which are normally only seen as distant possibilities or the plight of others."[2] When the person who gets sick is in her first few decades of life, the already-strange feeling of illness can feel extra strange. The researcher spoke with people who were experiencing rheumatological problems and were being diagnosed by doctors. "For the younger women," he writes, "it came as a profound shock to realise that arthritis could begin at their age." It felt like "premature ageing"—like an "abnormal" trajectory through one's twenties.

According to the developmental psychology volume of *The Handbook of Psychology*, many researchers suggest that "adolescents who are off time (earlier or later) in their pubertal development, with respect to peers, experience more stress than on-time adolescents."[3] Being off time may lead to a young person's not getting the usual social support or coping resources that those who are more on time receive. Similarly, in adulthood, when someone faces an event that is culturally expected to happen at a different time in the life cycle, according to the theories of Bernice Neugarten and Ravenna Helson, the event is perceived as more stressful, because it's inconsistent with societal expectations.[4]

When I visit Tracey Revenson, the professor of health psychology at Hunter College and the Graduate Center at the City University of New York, we talk about how important this concept is among young adults facing illness. After she read a series in the *New York Times* by Suleika Jaouad about having cancer in her twenties, Revenson tells me, she started to wonder. What are the unique stressors that young people face when coping with things like cancer? And how do those stressors differ in young women or other young adults of different socioeconomic groups?

While studying young adults who faced leukemia, Revenson found that those in their twenties and thirties kept coming back to this idea of off time. Whether they were talking about financial stress, fertility, relationships with their family, dating, or sex, age and identity kept coming up. When you've gone through serious illness in your twenties, thirties, or forties, often before your friends have, Revenson says, "you don't have peers that understand the experience and that you can discuss it with. It might be hard to find support. Illness at those ages is an off-time event." No matter what the stressor was, or the aspect of life these young adults discussed, she said, their peers simply didn't get it.

Many of the young adults in Revenson's study mentioned that in the hospital, they couldn't relate to anyone around them, either. The pediatric ward was filled with children and adolescents. Everyone else was decades older than they were.

In the scientific literature on cancer, Revenson says, studies lump together patients in broad age ranges, even though the age groups within those ranges are actually quite different. Especially in the breast cancer literature, she explains, researchers tend to draw a line at fifty because of menopause, and as a result, many studies refer to any patient under fifty as young. Those in their late forties, though, are in a different place than those in their twenties and thirties. In her own research, Revenson has been recommending that researchers need to untangle those age groups to understand what the specific developmental issues are and how the illness impacts the individuals' identity, careers, and social life. Emerging adults—those in their twenties—face unique circumstances. People this age are no longer adolescents, but are not completely adults, either. The idea of being between two stages, she says, dovetails with psychologist Jeffrey Arnett's theory of emerging adulthood. While some say those in their twenties are going through an extended adolescence, Arnett has argued that in today's world, this age is a different period, replete with different tasks that young adults are expected to accomplish. Young adult patients also face a type of uncertainty about things like career and fertility—issues unique to their age group.

Unfortunately, Revenson tells me, despite the unique challenges faced by young adults and, specifically, young women, there is little research on this group. Samantha Irby, the author who first documented her adventures with Crohn's disease on her blog, *Bitches Gotta Eat*, lists some of the highlights from an excruciating five days in the hospital: "being seen by [a] hot doctor in progressively gross condition, 'bathing' with 'fecal dissolving foam,' not having all of the fancy shit i need, getting woken up and stuck with needles every five minutes before i could even register what was happening, flashing the xray dude, TWICE, being disconnected from the universe, the $976,458,987,329 bill united healthcare is currently processing on my behalf, smelling weird," and other lovelies like "talking for half [an] hour with a nutritionist about corn pasta, and DIAPERS."[5]

She lists the many absurdly uncomfortable procedures she's had to go through—taboo things like having to "shit into this bowl contraption that hovered over the toilet water, then use the attached scoop and container to 'provide a sample.'" One of these is a CT scan. She writes, "I have had SEVEN of these goddamned things. SEVEN. Which means I have almost reached my lifetime limit for radiation exposure. And I AM THIRTY YEARS OLD."[6]

Like Irby, I sometimes want my peers to understand just how much I've been through before the age of thirty. When someone my age asks what kinds of health issues I've had, I say, "Well . . . the short version is thyroid cancer, hip surgery, and a scary rare anaphylaxis thing that sends me into anaphylactic shock for no reason and almost killed me three times. Oh, and somewhere in there, my dad also died." Then, if I see horror or shock in their eyes, I rush to say something flippant or funny with too much zest in my voice. "Really fun few years! But, yeah, tell me more about your screenplay!" I suddenly want them to see that even though I've been through a lot and feel old from it, I'm still their age: I'm totally fine.

The two aren't mutually exclusive, I've found, in the young women I've interviewed. They often want to honor the fact that they feel decades older than their years, while at the same time they want to fit in with friends and new acquaintances—even if sometimes that means pushing down their identity as sick or disabled. Being young often puts pressure on women to act chill, despite the difficult things they're going through.

Gender plays a role, too. As one woman who inherited a cancer-causing syndrome from her father tells me, "either directly or indirectly you get these messages from a very young age as a girl that compel you to keep your emotions in check. . . . There's all these expectations to *be cool*, like sleep with a guy and don't expect anything and *be cool*, don't be too emotional: *be cool*." Years of practice at remaining chill so as to not be "the crazy girl" or "the angry girl," she says, while dealing with her father's illness and now her own diagnosis, translated into an inability to communicate with her friends about health issues. "I definitely had practice suppressing my shit," she says.

———

On Samantha Kittle's blog about her post-brain-tumor life, she writes about close friends: "I was a groomslady in a wedding this weekend. I got to see my old friends from school. People who knew me before I became sick, which is something that is nigh impossible here in Chicago. I felt normal again. And realized that these people are extremely important to me, that I need to keep them closer . . . as I struggle through this whole being sick thing."[7]

That's something I think about a lot, too: people who knew me before I was sick versus everyone else from now on who will meet the "after-sickness" me. I suspect to my longtime friends I was more fun before, or less tainted by deathyness. Sometimes I just wish the friends I make today at a party can go back in time and see a glimpse of how I was before illness weighed me down. "There must be some way to integrate death into living, neither ignoring it nor giving in to it," Audre Lorde writes.[8] How do I live with this acute awareness of the unreliability of bodies, but not let on too much to my friends?

Actually, one longtime friend tells me, he thinks I seem pretty similar to how I was before. He doesn't perceive this heaviness that I think is following me around. That makes me wonder: Do I feel less light and sparkly inside, but present myself as light and sparkly around my friends?

Kittle describes her lighthearted weekend before her friend's wedding: giggling all morning with two of her friends, watching pig wrestling and public-access shows. Laughing nonstop, imitating the Men's Warehouse commercial while trying to get kicked out of a Men's Warehouse, laughing more, dancing at the party after the rehearsal dinner.

"The ceremony the next day had everyone in tears," she writes. "I was doing the weave tap to scratch under Erica"—the weave tap, meaning that she tapped on her brain-surgery-scar-covering wig, which she's named Erica, to alleviate the itch without messing it up. "I hoped I wasn't distracting anyone," she continues. "My chin was quivering from trying not to cry, I worried myself, unsure if I had taken my seizure meds that morning and feared that I was going to ruin the wedding by having a seizure right there in the Frank Lloyd Wright designed church."

In that one short summary of her weekend, I recognized a familiar turn: indulging in the responsible-ish version of hijinks, cracking up with your friends, feeling like a regular and carefree member of the group, part of some wonderful scene that's hilarious or moving or both, and then, in an instant, remembering your body, its protests, and worrying that a part of you that you can't control will suddenly ruin the moment.

In *Voices from the Shadows*, the 1983 book on women with disabilities, friendship comes up a lot, too. Gwyneth Ferguson Matthews's story goes back to December 1963, when she was sixteen and away at a junior college in Canada. Because the semester was ending soon, Matthews writes, she tried to ignore a high temperature and a doctor's diagnosis of flu. Incidentally, Matthews was herself planning on a career in medicine. She kept studying and began to sit for exams. While she was struggling with a French test, she writes, "a brutal headache hit me between the eyes. In minutes, it had travelled up my forehead, across my skull, and down to the back of my neck—a narrow band of agony."[9]

But Matthews kept ignoring it, focusing on her exams, until a few days later, when she collapsed.

After an agonizing period in the hospital, it became clear that Matthews's legs were paralyzed, and parts of her upper body, too.

"My friends poked their heads in occasionally," she writes, "asking if there was anything they could do." One time, she said that they could help her get out of bed. And so, she writes, "they put slippers on my unresponsive feet, slid them out of the blankets, and placed them on the floor. I grabbed the girls' arms, using the strength of desperation to try to stand. Useless."

Despite the complex emotions of being sixteen and realizing that she might not be able to use her legs to stand up the way she used to, Matthews performed for her friends. "I fell back, laughing hysterically," she writes, "convinced that an outsider would find the scene hilarious."

Later, she writes about coming to terms with the new way her body worked and the "turbulent feelings" she had. She felt tortured if she thought of riding a bicycle or dancing at high school sock hops.

"And," she writes, "I had another monumental problem to deal with: the abdication of my friends."

Once Matthews herself realized that, as she puts it, her disability was permanent, she found that her friends caught on—and stopped coming to see her. "Their visits," she writes, "formerly so regular, dwindled; by July, only one old faithful still came to see me. I felt deserted, and it was as if they had said, 'You're not good enough for us anymore.'"

A young woman Matthews interviews for her book had a similar experience. "A lot of my old friends haven't been to see me," the woman tells Matthews. "When I ask why so-and-so hasn't been, I hear, 'She doesn't want to see you in the wheelchair.' I sensed the ones that did come were uncomfortable. They always wanted to help, but they weren't sure what to do. It's like they've got their own lives and I'm not part of them anymore. It hurts."

When it comes to friends not understanding or trying to understand, the stories vary. Another of my journalism students, Paola, thanks me for the semester. It's the last day of class, and the other students are packing up. Paola tells me that she's graduating now, in the middle of the year, because she had to take off a semester earlier for health issues.

It was a pituitary tumor, she says. She'd started to have symptoms. Her hands were swelling, and, she thought, she was getting "really fat." But she also stopped getting her period. Something felt off. When she found out it was a tumor—not cancerous, but still dangerous, as it was causing her internal organs to swell as well—everything changed. She had to have surgery, through her nose, she says, to remove the tumor. She had to stay in the hospital for three weeks.

"They couldn't understand my pain," she says of her friends (and even her family members). She lost a best friend, she says, her best friend since fourth grade. Why?

Paola had told her best friend about the tumor and that she was going to be in the hospital. On the day that Paola was in the ICU, her best friend texted her: *Are you going out tonight?*

She was shocked by her best friend's callousness. The friend apparently had either chosen to ask about something superficial instead of texting about the surgery or had completely forgotten that her best friend was having an enormous medical procedure.

To make matters stranger, Paola says, her best friend's sister was an ENT nurse, a nurse who deals with ear, nose, and throat issues and who had actually helped with one of Paola's previous procedures. That sister texted helpful, supportive, and thoughtful things Paola's way—but Paola's best friend did not.

But the sister, who was older, was maybe more mature? I ask. It's possible, Paola says, that her best friend wasn't as mature as her sister, the nurse, but still. Her best friend should have texted her something like *Love you and thinking of you*—not a text about parties and bars.

You realize when you're sick who your friends really are, she says.

Many of the women I've met shared far more positive stories about their friends. Well, most of their friends. One young woman, a PhD candidate I met, had two friends who disappeared—twice. First, when she experienced what she calls a manic episode, both friends dropped off suddenly. Then, after she returned to her previous state of mental health, they came back to being her friend—only to do the same thing again and disappear when a thyroid syndrome, a stroke, and brain inflammation nearly killed her. Those two aside, the majority of her friends stayed by her. After seeing what she survived, they refer to her as a miracle.

These patterns came up with several women I've interviewed: a host of supportive, or at least trying-to-be-supportive friends, and then a few who either abruptly left the women's lives or slowly disappointed them, in sharp contrast to the friends who were there for the women all along.

But what does it even mean to *be there* for a friend who's going through health issues? For some women I've met, it can mean simply believing her when she says she's sick. It can mean remembering that your friend who's also twenty-two is getting ready for surgery and, no, can't come to the rager you're heading to at midnight. It can mean simply acknowledging the disparity between your experiences: *Hey, I know you're in the hospital right now. Sending you good thoughts. I'm heading out to meet Sana and Belinda at Matt's party. Wish you were here.* Rarely have I found young women who want a grand gesture of support, though some have been surprised and delighted when friends have made a huge effort.

More often, the way a friend can be there is simply to listen to you talk for more minutes than a nonsick person might. They could listen to how upsetting it is to have to rearrange your week for three doctors' appointments when you'd rather be getting work done. Or how frustrating it is to stay on the phone for an hour with your insurance company, only to find that the specialist you're finally able to see has absolutely nothing useful to say about your swollen joints or throbbing stomach. A friend could just listen when you say, *I spent the whole week in and out of doctors' offices, retelling my whole damn story and all the weird symptoms I've had the past few months, and all they did was order more tests and say they weren't sure.* Maybe after hearing this, they could try not to make it cheery somehow or immediately talk about the amazing film screening they went to while you were curled up in a fetal position. Sometimes, you just need the friend to say, *Oof. That sucks.*

As Samantha Irby puts it, she may joke a lot about her body, find the gallows humor in each absurd moment, but that doesn't mean she's gladly dealing with serious illness at a young age—or that she can always put on a smile or a laugh around her friends:

> i talk so much shit, but i really do get very sad when i'm counting out all of my pills and dragging economy-sized bags of adult diapers home on the train, when I'm ordering rubber underpants on the internet from websites that have pictures of smiling "active seniors" waving at me with their new comfort grip ultra absorbent poo pants and crinkly sheets that just wipe clean for incontinent elderly people who have accidents in bed, when the medical waste service comes to my apartment on mondays to exchange my shit cloths for clean ones. i heard that one of my friends recently described me as "bitter," and if it ever appears that way you know i don't mean it. bitter is one of those words with a fucking horrible connotation, and i promise you that isn't what i really am. i'm funny and everything, but what i really am is a thirty-one year old adult who spends a lot of time sick and drugged and diapered. so pardon me if I'm not a ray of sunshine 100% of the goddamned time.[10]

Irby gets at one of the paradoxes of being young and sick. On the one hand, you're trying to seem just dandy around your friends and show them the funny and carefree side of yourself that young people might expect of you. On the other, being sick isn't all lightness and air, and sometimes, whether you're around friends or strangers, you actually need your health issue to be more visible or taken seriously. You need others to recognize that part of your light mood might be real, but that when you're tired of your illness or in pain, the facade may wear away.

A few summers ago, I was in Jackson, Mississippi, on a cross-country train trip. During a tour of the state capitol building, a volunteer explained the term *scagliola*. It's the technique of taking a piece of plaster and some glues and dyes and painstakingly decorating it with faux-marble veins so that it looks like solid stone.

The other people on the tour spoke in low, awestruck voices about the unbelievable simulacrum, how much the building's pillars looked like marble, even though, as the tour guide said, the material needed upkeep for the facade to work. I was impressed, too, though I felt a weird sense of pride about detecting that something looked off about it.

Oh, I realized. I'm the scagliola.

Because I am young, and because I do want to seem buoyant when I can, I'm constantly masked. Sometimes by choice, other times by default because of how my body appears, I'm painted over to look like something more solid. And so people find it hard to believe that underneath I am crumbling plaster.

After my second hip surgery and the searing pain of even the slightest movement, I spent six or so weeks trying to get off crutches, feeling both the relief of not using my tendons that had been cut and the dread that every time I went outside, I was That Girl on Crutches.

Finally, after a few too-early attempts to walk without them, including my Census Bureau experience, I was done with the crutches. I could—carefully, my physical therapist said—go outside and take some short walks on my own. My friend Sarah was visiting all the way from Singapore that week, so naturally I interpreted "carefully" as I wished. Instead of walking ten blocks and giving my still-healing hip a rest, I decided that Sarah and I would tour some museums whose exhibits she wanted to see, traipse about clothing stores she couldn't access in Singapore, and stroll around till we found a good restaurant for lunch.

*Tour*, *traipse*, and *stroll* were not supposed to be part of my body's vocabulary yet. After Sarah and I walked around the Whitney, I felt the familiar heat up my neck, the feeling that came with realizing I'd overused my body, pretended it worked as well as it looked when it did not. It's similar to the heat rushing up my neck after I've embarrassed myself at a party or, when I was younger, after I learned that I had missed an entire page on a math test an hour after handing it in. It's knowing I did something wrong and realizing it too late.

Sooo, my hip is kind of hurting a lot and I think I need to take the bus, I told Sarah. I said it tentatively. Meanwhile, my hip was in excruciating, I-shouldn't-have-walked-through-an-entire-museum pain, but to my friend, I wanted it to seem only "kind of" hurting. And I didn't want to be the fun-spoiler, the one who told a visitor from halfway across the earth that we couldn't wander, as she loves to do, and pop into stores on a whim, but had to take the boring bus.

I mean, maybe I could walk a little longer, I said, maybe a few more blocks. I was always trying to minimize my difference and seem like just any twentysomething. I was always pushing my hurt body past the initial feeling of pain and then the second more overwhelming wall of pain so I could be a "regular" young person who can walk and hang out.

When we finally got on the bus, Sarah and I dipped our Metro-Cards and then stood for a moment as the bus lurched forward again. I realized the situation was untenable: each time the bus swung left or right or suddenly gained speed, I couldn't stabilize myself and almost fell. The hip, I'd learned, though we tend to think of it in the context of an older person's problems, can easily destabilize if all its complex parts aren't working together properly or are weak. The way buses lurch and stop and bang through potholes and dart around taxis meant repeated stabs of pain and the inability to stand up. So despite having learned as a kid that the seats in the very front were for the elderly, disabled, or pregnant, and despite my refusal to categorize myself as having any disability whatsoever and feeling a swell of guilt since my joint problems seemed at the time to be temporary, I sat down.

And then, a woman with white hair screamed at me.

"You shouldn't sit there!" she yelled. "That's for people my age!"

"Oh," I said. "I know I look young, but I actually just had hip surgery."

"It's not for people your age!" she shouted. "You're healthy!"

"But . . . I just had hip surgery," I said. "I need to sit. I can't stand up while the bus is jerking around."

The woman gave me a look of malice. She didn't stop chastising me until finally another older woman in the section said something like, "She said she had surgery. Let her sit."

*But you're too young.* The line that many of us hear again and again. But you're too young to have cancer. But you're too young to have arthritis. My grandma had hip surgery and she's eighty. You're healthy! Look at you! Aren't you too young?

Just this week, I've heard the line twice. I'd told one of my favorite doctors that while traveling a few years ago in Singapore (for

Sarah-of-the-traipsing's wedding) with terrifyingly bad ankle pain that stopped me from frolicking around the city, I'd gone to a doctor there and had gotten some patches from him after he'd ruled out every other medication. He was worried about all my allergies and unusual reactions to anti-inflammatories and had told me that although the patches weren't usually for joint problems, he thought they would work. I'd plunked down more than a hundred dollars for a small box of the cooling, analgesic-coated rectangles and was thrilled as soon as I pasted one to my ankle.

Now, back in New York, I'd told the doctor about the patches, the way they eased joint pain and even seemed to temporarily heal the ankle problem without causing any other bizarre reaction in my body. "Lidocaine patches?" she'd said. "I usually prescribe those to my old people, but, huh, that makes sense for you. I'll have to keep that in mind for other young patients. I'd never thought about it! Huh. Lidocaine!"

This is a doctor I adore and whom I've been seeing for almost a decade. I'm sure my cheek twitched a little when she made the point about how the lidocaine patches were for old people, but I appreciated that she decided to consider prescribing them in the future to people who could benefit from them, regardless of age. I tucked the prescription into my wallet to remember to bring it to the pharmacy.

"We have these in stock," my pharmacist said later that day. He looked at me. "You're too *young* for lidocaine patches."

For a second, I wanted to give him the benefit of the doubt: that he was an informed pharmacist and good at his job and had actually caught something my doctor had done wrong. Maybe I was, in fact, too young and would somehow cause a problem by using them. But no, I realized. It was the same thing as always. Someone telling me that I'm too young for health problems, despite the overwhelming evidence that those health problems had found me in my twenties and snuggled right in.

It may not seem like a big deal to people who haven't heard the line. Maybe it sounds like a compliment, *You're too young*, something to show that you look youthful and vibrant and all. Maybe it's just a refrain I should learn to ignore. But when I talk with other young women who hear it over and over again, they too roll their eyes and look upset. We do feel that we got sick too soon, decades before we'd expected to feel our bodies break down. But if there were truly such a thing as too young to be sick, then we wouldn't be sick. And we are.

Jen, the one who's had men on the street curse at her and her health issues and who had male partners tell her she deserved the response, framed the street harassment incident as one about older men in particular. In general, she says, she's had a lot of people older than her tell her, "You're too young to be sick," or, "You look too good to be sick." It's eerie to hear her say word for word what people have told me.

Those who are a few decades older than her, she says, are largely the ones who don't believe her about her own body. She remembers a time when she was leaning heavily on her cane, with a swollen foot. A woman nearby seemed to tell from Jen's face that she was about to ask for a seat. She looked Jen up and down, made a derisive noise, and looked the other way.

We talk about how strange it is—because in these moments, her disability isn't even invisible. She's using a mobility aid. She's had the interactions on buses in Seattle, too, she says, where she grew up: bus drivers who wouldn't lower the steps for her, even though they would for an older person.

"Take a hint," Jen says. "If I'm on crutches and I have my foot in a boot, like, take a hint."

I tell her I've had the same thing happen with an (older, male) bus driver in New York. The man saw that I was on crutches. And he refused to lower the steps. He just stared at me, watched me struggle. When I asked him to lower the bus, he continued to refuse, even though I was visibly using crutches. He looked me right in the eye and told me I didn't need it.

When people say, "You're too young," they're telling people like Jen and me that we must be making up our pain, our surgeries. But they're also ignoring that, statistically, many, many young people have joint problems, cancer, or autoimmune issues. What the phrase *too young* really conveys, then, isn't fact, but our culture's expectation that health issues are for only certain demographics, that youth is carefree.

As Suleika Jaouad writes in her *New York Times* column about being a twentysomething woman with leukemia, having a life-threatening disease this early in young adulthood "carries a special set of psychological and social challenges. It defies our very definition of what ought to be. Youth and health are supposed to be synonymous. If only I could sue my body for breach of contract with the natural order of things."[11]

Cancer, she continues, "magnifies the in-betweenness of young adulthood: You're not a child anymore, yet you're not fully ready to live in the adult world, either." Jaouad, like other women, and like me, found herself back in her childhood bedroom while going through treatment. She had to rely on her parents for help, but at the same time, she was growing up faster than her same-age friends who had no health issues.

And, she writes, with cancer in particular, "young adults might just be oncology's 'tweens'—too old for the pediatric cancer floor but equally out of place in an adult oncology unit. I'm not suggesting that it's worse to be young and sick, but rather that young adults with cancer are a less visible demographic, swept up in the mix of adult cancer statistics."

———

A month or so after doctors revived me from anaphylaxis and brought me back into the world of regular post-college life—or what we think that's supposed to be—it was impossible to be the person my friends expected. One night, I decide that it's time to make myself "normal" again. I agree to go to a party. The idea is to make myself go out and be the kind of person who's all about hanging and listening to music and meeting new people and just being. But I can't stop double-checking for the epinephrine injectors in my bag or thinking about where the nearest emergency room is as a friend's boyfriend drives us to Brooklyn. It is unusual to be in a car—we almost always take the train everywhere—but in some ways it is a relief to ride above ground and not on the subway. Whenever the train stands still in the tunnel, my mind flashes back to the emergency room. Even with an EpiPen plunged perfectly through my jeans to my thigh, even if a stranger can do it correctly, hold the needle in for ten seconds straight to deliver the medicine, even if they figure it out before I completely stop breathing, what are the odds that I'll get above ground from the subway tunnel in time? What are the odds that the pen will even work right, that I won't die right there on the R train, collapse as I did three weeks before?

So I am grateful for the car, even if I usually prefer the subway. The car is closer to hospitals, and for that reason alone, it makes my foray back into nightlife less frightening.

In the car, though, my friend starts to ask what exactly the deal is with this weird allergy-testing diet I'm now on. Why can I only eat the same few things every day? Do doctors really think I have a new fatal food allergy and that that's why I went into anaphylaxis?

Or maybe I'm remembering wrong. Maybe she wasn't asking, and maybe I started telling her what I'd been going through since the hospital, how every bite of a new food could be deadly.

We don't know yet, I say, because if it is a new food allergy that tried to strangle me from the inside out, then it could really be anything. The culprit could be the sesame seeds on the bread I ate or the thyme that was sprinkled on the rice. It could be peppercorns. It could be what's at the party tonight.

My friend asks what I'm up to—which food is next on my list to try. I'm allowed one new food every two days, no spices or sauces. One item, plain, that I've always been able to eat but now have to test as if it's arsenic or a bomb. I tell her I want to reintroduce cheese, maybe goat cheese, maybe cheddar. I think the strain in my voice is evident. As my friend or just as a person, either way, she can probably detect my fear when I talk. It's not a small thing to try a new cheese when the cheese might kill you. But she—my friend—makes it a joke. Maybe to impress her boyfriend, maybe because she just can't understand it. I don't know why, but she does.

"Uh-oh, what if we slip you some blue cheese tonight and you're not ready for it yet!" she snorts. "What if you try Swiss before you're supposed to!" She's laughing, a mean laugh. It is only now, years later, that I realize she wasn't mean in her mind, but probably trying to lighten up a heavy conversation about how her friend had almost died. But in that car, I am throat-sore now, I feel the hoarseness that always gives me away before a cry. She hears nothing. And then her boyfriend chimes in.

"Ha!" he says. "You're totally scared of goat cheese. That's crazy."

At this point, I use all my strength to harness the muscles that want to cry. I am already a killjoy on the way to a party, talking about the way I almost died. I am the weirdo here. I am the one taking my friends to a place that twenty-two-year-olds don't want to go. I try to muster a laugh, but it comes out forced. I try instead to tell them to stop. But how do you plead with a good friend who should know to stop being flippant about your throat closing up? How do you say, *Uh, Eve, it isn't funny to talk about the goat cheese or gang up on me with your boyfriend when neither of you knows what it's like to nearly die and come back. It isn't okay to make me feel stupid for my fear when the doctor last week says he's not sure how I survived?*

I am angry and hurt, and more than that, I am scared. If your friends won't protect you or see they're hurting you, then who are your friends?

But in hindsight, again, they were probably trying to smooth over a terrifying, unknowable thing. In general, I do like joking about my health. Actually, much of the time, gallows humor is my only coping mechanism, and I'm the one making the jokes. The difference this time is that I have just narrowly escaped dying, and I don't know when the mystery illness will strike again. I'm usually self-deprecating to a fault. I make fun of myself and my circumstances often, and maybe my friend is used to that version of me. I want to still be that version of myself, to be in the we're-having-fun-and-about-to-be-at-a-party mode, but in this moment, I can't be. This is too raw and too still-happening to make light of. *Too soon*, as the joke goes, but actually, not jokingly, too soon. I stare out the car window and try not to cry.

"When people want to talk about their fears, they want to talk about their fears, not to be told, quite blatantly, that their fears are imaginary," writes Deborah Orr in a piece for the *Guardian* called "10 Things Not to Say to Someone When They're Ill."[12] When she was diagnosed with cancer, Orr writes, she needed to talk about how much she dreaded becoming bald from the treatment. She didn't want to hear people tell her there was nothing to worry about; she brought it up precisely because she needed to vent. To those of us going through something tough that our peers may not be able to relate to, sometimes we just need to talk it out. And if we cherish our friends and love to hang out with them, I've found, it can be hard to say, "Actually, can you just let me vent for a minute about this, 'cause it'll make me feel a little less shitty about my week going to all these doctors?" It feels stilted, and not fun, to say something like that when your friends usually think of you as someone lighthearted. It's hard when you're young to interrupt the usual banter with your heaviness.

And then there are the empty sentiments, too. Friends and acquaintances can be extremely well-meaning, I've realized, and still say something quite off-tone. I have grown to understand that people often do mean well. But when they're confronted with someone they care about having a health issue or someone's health issue reminding them of their own mortality, they just don't know what to say. Perhaps that's why a series of illness greeting cards went viral a few years ago. Created by a woman named Emily McDowell, who went through stage 3 Hodgkin's lymphoma at age twenty-four, the cards are a response to the type of unhelpful things people sometimes say.[13]

"When life gives you lemons," one card reads, "I won't tell you a story about my cousin's friend who died of lemons." Another reads, "Please let me be the first to punch the next person who tells you everything happens for a reason," and then, in small letters below, "I'm sorry you're going through this." There are also quieter ones that probably resonate with a lot of people, including the people on the card-giving end: "You're not a burden. You're a human," and, "I'm really sorry I haven't been in touch. I didn't know what to say."[14]

"The most difficult part of my illness," McDowell writes on her card company's blog, "wasn't losing my hair, or being erroneously called 'sir' by Starbucks baristas, or sickness from chemo. It was the loneliness and isolation I felt when many of my close friends and family members disappeared because they didn't know what to say, or said the absolute wrong thing without realizing it."[15] With the cards, she hopes to give people a way to communicate about what illness is like in a real way, to help well-meaning friends actually say something helpful.

Vita was living in Oakland when she was diagnosed with MS. She had already planned a trip to Los Angeles with some of her good friends before she learned she needed a spinal tap. When she went to have it done, a resident inserted the needle in her back ten times until it finally became clear that the procedure wasn't working. After a doctor arrived and took over, Vita had to endure two more insertions before the procedure was done right. And the side effects of the spinal tap meant that Vita, who determinedly went on this trip with her friends, was unable to walk more than a few steps without lying down. She would walk, lie down, walk a few more steps, lie down, and occasionally throw up in the bushes while her friends enjoyed the beach.

Later, with the same group of good friends from college, Vita was on a trip abroad. They were preparing to climb a volcano the following day. Then Vita's left leg went numb. She decided to climb the volcano anyway, even though her nerves couldn't sense what was under her feet. She relied on her other leg to drag her up the volcano. The next day, her body was in such rough shape that her friends had to help cart her around.

Other friends did fall away. "I think a lot of people with illness experience this exodus," she says. These are people who exit your life because for whatever reason, they can't deal with it. She had friends who told her they couldn't be around her and her MS. Other friends said it reminded them of something else, or someone else who was ill, and they just didn't want to be around illness. Or they didn't want to tough it out when things got rough.

Vita says she was used to being the kind of friend who people came to for emotional support. Suddenly, she needed some support, and she wasn't comfortable asking for it.

Her friends from the beach and volcano trips are still around, she says. She lost friends, but not the close ones. It definitely still hurt, she tells me, but it would have been devastating had the friends who ditched her been among her closest.

One friend who couldn't handle it was Vita's roommate. She was cold toward Vita any time Vita mentioned the diagnosis process. But because the roommate's mother had been sick for much of her life, Vita understood that the friend lacked the emotional capacity to now watch another person go through a diagnosis.

It's frustrating, she says, that most people have no clue what she's going through and make very little effort to understand what it's like. Then their reaction, she says, is often to either step away or be overly doting and weird about it, or treat you like you're four. Still, she understands that people have trouble dealing with health issues. Now that the emotional hurt has subsided for Vita, she and the former roommate are, several years later, rekindling their friendship.

In terms of community, Vita tends to hang out in radical, queer, people-of-color spaces. And yet, she says, even though she finds solidarity about other things in these communities, she also finds herself wishing these spaces were sick. Folks can be radical or can relate to her about being a woman of color, but they can't relate to her about illness. So to get that kind of community and understanding, she says she usually has to go to a white and nonradical place, where she doesn't feel at home, either. In her own circles, she's used to people of color joking about race and pain and oppression in their lives as a coping mechanism—gallows humor. And yet, when she makes the same kind of jokes about illness, they don't get it. They clam up.

Eileen, the patient navigator, tells me how it worked for her when she had breast cancer at thirty-four—how friendship and illness and being young intersected.

"Everybody around me was totally healthy," she says. "I had friends whose *mothers* had breast cancer, but never [anyone] my age at all. There was nobody I could really identify with from my friends at all. All of us were sort of at the stage where we were all having little babies, so we experienced that together. But in this, I was all by myself. I should say that my friends were actually extremely supportive even though they could not identify with the hugeness of having cancer."

A couple of close friends showed up at Eileen's doorstep, unannounced. Without telling her, they'd bought plane tickets and flown in from faraway states the moment they'd heard her bad news. That's being there, I suppose, in a physical sense.

Still, throughout the ten months of her diagnosis, surgeries, and chemotherapy, Eileen felt a lot older than her friends. Everyone was posting pictures of themselves. "You would see people going out, or traveling," she says. She was just trying to get through treatment. She made new friends in a spiritually oriented church that she joined, and, she says, "my friends started becoming older. The people I was around were in their fifties and sixties"—her mom's age. Although she couldn't relate to the older volunteers at the hospital or the older women in the cancer support groups, she did still gravitate toward her elders.

Other women describe the same sensibility. One twenty-five-year-old with chronic health issues writes, "I do not relate at all to people my age, I never have. I have always felt so much more comfortable in the company of older people." The main reason, she writes, is that "older people know what it is like to have your body fail you. They have been through a lot over the course of their entire lives, while we chronically ill people have gone through a lot in the course of a few years."[16]

Another young woman I interview talks about how her health issues chafe against her friendships in a few ways that are unique to her identity. Lucy, who introduces herself to me by e-mail as "a trans Latina with depression and anxiety disorders" and who's also queer, writes, "My mental health, sadly, and frustratingly, sometimes really affects my friendships. I don't want to use it as an excuse, it's not that, I need to be responsible for my behavior. Sometimes though, I fall into bad pits of depression and I'm bad at staying in touch with my friends. I have friends all over the country, so if I'm not putting in work to stay in contact with them, it hurts the relationship."

It sounds to me like Lucy is beating herself up over something that's not really her fault. Then again, maybe she truly does fall off the map when her health issues hit, and maybe it's healthy to hold herself accountable. But it sounds like she's judging herself harshly.

"I also deal with a lot of suicidal ideation," she writes, "and I deal with self-harm, and I have very, very few friends I can talk to about that. By very few, I mean one. Some of my friends I'm afraid to tell, some struggle with similar things and would be triggered, some have told me that it's too stressful for them to be a person I talk to about those things."

Ah, I think. Here's yet another young woman trying to seem *totally fine* to her friends—at least, the ones she's afraid to tell. Then, from the ones she has told, she's gotten feedback that her health issues are too overwhelming for them to hear about.

"I understand, though," she says of the latter. "It takes a lot of strength and work to be there for me when I'm going through bad depressive spells. I want to be able to be the best friend I can, and often I feel like I can't because of my depression."

I ask Lucy about that one friend whom she can actually open up to about her health. Is it a friend who just happens to have a lot of capacity for "holding space," as people put it—for listening and being present even when someone tells you something hard to deal with? Or is it more because this friend has gone through similar mental health issues and so can relate firsthand?

Perhaps not surprisingly, this friend has similar hard things in her life, too. She is, Lucy writes, "a queer Latina, just like me," who deals with mental health issues around depression and self-harm. The friend is cisgender, not trans, Lucy writes. "But we're able to relate on a ton of stuff. It's really nice to have someone who can relate and really understands what helps and what doesn't."

What still jumps out, though, is how much Lucy feels like she's a burden to every other friend but this one.

"Do you think that being trans in a transphobic world teaches you to feel already like a 'burden' to your peers," I ask, "or less of a 'good' or 'easy' friend to others—again, just because of internalized transphobic cultural shit—and that having mental health stuff on top of that makes you extra worried about being a 'difficult' friend?" In my e-mail, I tell her, "You definitely sound like you're beating yourself up about it, and so I wonder if part of it is already having an identity that transphobic society has labeled as 'difficult.'"

In other words, has our culture taught Lucy that as a trans woman, she already has to apologize for herself to begin with, and that her health issues only add to that? Or, I ask, "do you think that whether or not you were trans, you would still feel a bit like a burden to friends when you were having mental health stuff?"

Her answer surprises me a bit.

"I do internalize a lot of transphobia and stuff," she writes, "and I often worry that if I talk to my cis friends about certain things, they'll see me as a guy."

The issue, then, is that Lucy is worried she is betraying some kind of "maleness" in her behavior when she's depressed. She explains a little more about her fear that friends will see her this way.

"Like, if I talk about relationships or sex or anything like that," she writes, "I'm really afraid they will [think I'm like a man]. I'm just afraid that when I act like a bad friend because of my depression, my friends will think that I'm acting like a guy. Growing up I saw every way that guys acted and I hated it and couldn't relate to it. I created extreme rules about how boys act and when I do anything close to that, I beat myself up about it and I assume that my friends will too." When her mental health issues crop up, she tells me, "when I get angry or I'm a bad listener or I'm selfish, those are things I associate with men."

On the one hand, I'm not surprised that Lucy polices her own gender presentation. It's something commonly discussed among trans women and trans men who want to be taken seriously as women or men, respectively, and it's something that even those of us who are cisgender do all the time, consciously and subconsciously. As a woman who's a bit genderqueer, I find that Lucy's talk of "extreme rules" about how different genders are supposed to act resonates with some of my experiences, too. But in Lucy's case, the stakes are much higher. Her health issues not only are difficult to deal with internally, but also make her worry that friends will "catch" her being male, even though she's a woman who faces discrimination and violence just for being trans.

———

I ask Sophie, the scientist who was born with HIV, if she, like me, sometimes becomes friends with someone and then later finds out that the person has also dealt with mortality at a young age. She has noticed a similar trend. Sophie calls herself a big mouth, affectionately. When she was a kid, she says, her mother impressed on her that about this one thing—Sophie's health—not everyone would understand. Now, as an adult, she has a group of friends who all have serious health issues. "So," she says, "we call each other the misfits."

When unsuspecting peers, ones who don't know Sophie has HIV, make thoughtless or rude jokes about people with the virus in Sophie's presence, her other friends, those who are in the know, change the topic. They maneuver the conversation in a different direction to stop the thoughtless comments without outing Sophie.

"All my life, I've heard the jokes," Sophie says. "All my life, I've sat and listened, and I've had to be the smiley person, or I've had to be the educated person. And I've just listened to their jokes."

Her peers have often been taken aback when she says she's HIV positive. "Stop lying," a fellow student in a medical class once told her. The person had a preconception of what someone with the virus looks like and didn't believe that Sophie could be that person. Another line that Sophie is tired of hearing is, "You're not what I expect."

Although the comments may change slightly, depending on the person or the illness, many women who have less visible health issues or disabilities have heard a version of the same. There's the favorite line: "But you're too young." And then, there's that bromide's hollower, more sexist cousin, one I've heard too many times: "Well, at least you're thin!"

*Right*, I always want to say. *I'm so glad I look thin while healing from a scalpel to my neck.*

Many of the young women I've interviewed have seen adults, and especially adults older than they are, refuse to believe that they are ill. I've encountered the same. And while we're trying to seem totally fine with our peers much of the time, our feelings change when people straight-up don't believe us. We want people—we need people—to recognize that our bodies are doing some difficult things underneath our youthful exterior. That we're not making up being on crutches. We do need the bus to be lowered, or we can't get on board.

Even when people do believe a young woman who says she's just been through major surgery or treatment, they often think of her as an outlier. In fact, young women are, statistically, the primary demographic for many major illnesses.

As NIH reports, autoimmune diseases—"a group of more than 80 chronic and often disabling illnesses that develop when underlying defects in the immune system lead the body to attack its own organs, tissues, and cells"—occur nearly 80 percent of the time in women.[17] Some diseases emerge in women far more than they do in men. For example, a whopping 90 percent of lupus cases occur in women. And when it comes to age, many of these conditions—for instance, multiple sclerosis—occur more in female patients than they do in males and tend to strike when women are young, in their twenties and thirties. Breast cancer, meanwhile, tends to be more aggressive in younger than in older women and flings hundreds of thousands of young women each year into unexpected crises of body image and fertility.

Because our culture generally overlooks young adults with cancer, a few organizations have emerged to support this demographic. Stupid Cancer, for instance, is a nonprofit focused on cancer in young adults, which it defines as ages fifteen through thirty-nine. This age group, the website says, is overlooked, "with 72,000 new diagnoses each year. That's one every eight minutes. *This is not OK!* This neglected group—now millions strong—has limited resources, inadequate support, and, more importantly, a lack of awareness and understanding from the community around them."[18] Another group, called First Descents, whose happy hour I once attended, "provides life-changing outdoor adventures for young adults (ages 18–39) impacted by cancer." An organization called the Samfund, a grant-making nonprofit for young people who have been through cancer, was founded by a woman who had the disease at a young age and realized how much it costs, emotionally and financially, for those who are just starting out as adults. There's also the Young Survival Coalition, for young women with breast cancer. And there's Lacuna Loft, a nonprofit that connects young adult cancer survivors around the world.[19]

But there are many serious illnesses that affect young women and, in particular, young women of color disproportionately, even if cancer tends to be a bit more in the public consciousness. Lupus, for instance, disproportionately affects African American, Asian American, Latinx, and Native American women.[20] And research out of Emory University found that among those who are diagnosed, African American women present with the disease younger and with more complications.[21] The study's principal investigator, S. Sam Lim, associate professor in the Division of Rheumatology, says, "Black women had very high rates of lupus, with an incidence rate in Georgia nearly three times higher than that for white women, with significantly high rates in the 30–39 age group . . . These are young women in the prime of their careers, family and fertility. This means a severely compromised future with a disease that waxes and wanes, affecting every aspect of daily living for the rest of their lives."[22]

Lupus, cancer, multiple sclerosis—they're just a few of the issues that young women face silently, without sufficient support, as the rest of their communities tell them they're too youthful-looking to be sick.

While women of all ages feel pressure to look and act a certain way, those in their first few decades are expected to be at their most vivacious. Their bodies, they know, are a kind of "public project," as historian Joan Jacobs Brumberg puts it in *The Body Project: An Intimate History of American Girls*.[23] Another woman describes it this way for an essay in the *Rumpus*: "As a woman, I am used to the fact that what I look like is considered to be either my greatest asset or saddest failure. And as a physically disabled woman, I am a sad afterthought in a society where women's bodies make up a large portion of their value."[24]

Being scrutinized for your physical appearance is hard enough as a woman in good health. Suddenly, your body feels even more exposed once it begins what we perceive as an early decline. We tend to equate young with healthy and old with infirm. We are wary of a twenty-year-old with joint inflammation or a cane or a crutch, but praise a seventy-year-old who has "succeeded" in staying arthritis-free.

Some women with cancer or other health issues feel they must defend themselves from curious outsiders who either don't believe them or who wonder what they did wrong. *Diagnosed even though I worked out and ate broccoli* is a line I've heard more than once.

A 2012 study in the *Journal of Affective Disorders* found that women were significantly more likely than men were to have anxiety and depression after cancer diagnosis and that, for certain types of cancers, younger women were especially in emotional distress. The study also found that in general, age and emotional distress were inversely related. When participants were older, they were less anxious and stressed. When they were younger, they reported more anxiety.[25]

And then there are the young women who are so used to their bodies working the way we expect young bodies to work that, in the days leading up to their diagnosis, their symptoms don't worry them. They assume they must be fine.

Erin, a white, cisgender woman who's in her mid-forties when I meet her, tells me her story. She went abroad during her junior year of high school, she says, and when she came back, she stayed with her sister, who was in Florida.

"I was gorgeous in the way that sixteen- or seventeen-year-olds are," she says. "Tan, good butt, long hair." She and her sister, who was then twenty-two, spent a lot of their time at the beach.

Then Erin started to notice strange bruises. She figured they were from the bumpy rides on the days her sister had been teaching her to drive. One morning, she woke up with blood all over her mouth. It was strange, but it registered as only slightly worrisome. After all, she was young, and it was summer. She and her sister got dressed for the beach—bikinis, sunscreen, sunglasses. They were ready for the ocean but decide to stop at a local doctor on the way. The idea was to get the symptoms checked out, then head to the sand.

But the doctor told Erin she needed to go to the hospital. He didn't explain why. Erin and her sister, still in their bikinis, didn't understand what was going on, but they did as he said.

The hospital gave Erin platelets and said something about her bone marrow. She'd heard about bone marrow before, because a little girl she'd heard about had needed it—and that girl had leukemia.

Erin realized what might be happening, but the doctors at the hospital didn't explain what was going on. They prodded her, then told her to fly home to Massachusetts and go straight to her parents. Trying to comprehend what was happening, Erin flew home, still with her bikini and beach bag and sunglasses for a day she had assumed would be warm and carefree. Her parents brought her to another hospital right away, where Erin got the news: she did have leukemia, and the odds of her surviving were extremely low. She ended up living through it. But that day, she emphasizes, was supposed to be all ocean and sun and being young.

This was in the mid-1980s. Erin had heard of people dying from leukemia, but not of them surviving it. After two rounds of chemotherapy, she says, she became so sick that she was taken to the ICU. Although she now knows that she was there for forty-nine days, it felt like only four or five. A blur. She deteriorated so much that doctors eventually told her family that she was near death and that the only thing they could do was experimental: a last-ditch effort to try to get her to live past the next day or two. So, at the doctors' request, her parents found people who were willing to donate platelets—platelets that could either save her or kill her.

Once she was stabilized, Erin says, friends came to visit. She was hooked up to all kinds of monitors, she remembers, and when the boys she was friends with—they were a few years older and in college—came to visit, they took turns going into her room to see which of them made her heart beat faster. That was sweet of them, she thinks now. At the time, she remembers feeling she looked awful: emaciated, ashen, bald, with a bloated stomach, no longer that gorgeous late teen with great hair. The first time she got home and looked in the mirror, she sobbed.

After another stay in the hospital, she was eventually allowed to go back to class, a boarding school where she was "a scholarship kid." The other students knew why she looked strange, she says, but she still wanted to cover it up. So she wore a wig. At some point, her dorm did a skit in which the younger girls imitated the seniors, and a girl from a younger grade snatched Erin's wig off her head and put it on to do an impression.

It was funny and sweet, Erin says. She remembers it fondly. But she still wasn't ready for anyone outside of that small group of girls to see her bald.

Even with the wig on, though, she stood out. She'd gone from around 135 pounds to just 85. That on its own would be enough. But in addition, she'd needed a port—a device that doctors implant just below the skin so that chemotherapy medicines and other fluids can be easily pumped into the patient's bloodstream. The doctors had given her a choice: a port that would sit between her breasts or one that would be a bit more difficult, near her underarm. Because she didn't want something protruding from between her breasts, she opted for the more difficult port. But she was so skinny, she says, that even the more hidden port stuck out from her skeletal figure.

Although she'd missed classes while in the ICU, Erin had applied and been accepted into college already. Her parents fought with her high school to let her graduate. As a first-year college student the next year and with her leukemia now in remission, she tried to seem like any other young woman there. Her natural hair color, a very dark brown, had begun to grow back in as light blonde, she says, so people called it frosted and thought she'd done it on purpose. They figured she had cut it short and bleached it like Annie Lennox, the singer who was popular at the time and known for her androgynous style. Erin didn't tell the other students what really drove the new look.

While hiding a huge experience you've just been through, I've learned, does let you "pass" as someone who is just fine, doing so can also put great pressure on you. If you don't tell anyone about your health or how close you came to not being here anymore, then nobody knows to support you. Plus, for young women who, like Erin, are committed to keeping their health trials to themselves, small talk becomes something you have to gingerly step through without giving yourself away. An innocent question from a classmate—"Love the hair! Where'd you get it done?"—suddenly seems impossible to answer. If you don't let on, the person has no idea that as you say, "Aw, thanks!" and figure out what to say next, your mind is back in the chemo suite.

# PART 4

# Why Don't They Believe Me? or the Case of the Lady Lab Rat

After Brenda experienced a year of neurological symptoms, her primary doctor suggested she see a neurologist. And then, she says, "the first neuro asked if I was making it up."

Brenda, then twenty-eight and working in politics, had experienced a slowing down of her left limbs, then her right. She'd been running marathons, and the trainer she ran with had noticed her gait changing. But the doctor didn't believe it was real.

"I can still recall his exact wording," she says. "'Is it possible that these symptoms are not actually there? Could it be a mental health issue?'"

At that, she says, "I remember being shocked and stunned. And saying something like, 'No, I'm not inventing this.'" She left the appointment, went to her car, and cried.

I ask if she ever returned to him or immediately saw a second neurologist. I explain that I'm asking because sometimes, even when doctors makes you feel awful or do something unprofessional or bigoted, they're specialists or they're "the experts," and you think you still need them for your health issue.

"Oh heck no!" she says. "I can still picture him and will never forget his name. I laugh because his last name—while spelled differently—is the Spanish word for stupid." She continues, "I'm fortunate that I have incredible health insurance through my employer and never went back to see him."

"Man. Makes my blood boil hearing that, even second hand," I say. I ask if this interaction with the first neurologist made her worried about the next.

It was a top university hospital, she says. "I figured that if they thought I was making it up, then I had to reevaluate. But in my heart, I knew I wasn't making this up."

Hold on a minute, I think, when I hear Brenda's response. If it hadn't been for this doctor accusing her of making it all up, it sounds as if she would never have started wondering about the idea of making it up in the first place. She knew that her symptoms were real. Her trainer did. Her primary doctor seemed to as well. But this reaction from the specialist had made her question herself, even though she'd had a year of progressive neurological symptoms.

"Correct," she says. "I had never entertained the idea of my making it up; it had never crossed my mind. My primary doctor had never questioned it. My trainer knew something was off. No one else had ever brought it up." And then: "It certainly made me question my state of mind. I started to see a psychologist—just to make sure."

This one physician had done all that, in one appointment. And it has happened to other women, too.[1] The doctor has power and authority, qualities that make it easy to start questioning yourself. But Brenda knew this wasn't the way it should have gone. Within a few days, she contacted the hospital where the doctor was based and told them the story. She never heard back. It makes her furious to think that he's still there, at the same hospital, seeing patients.

Now, several years later, Brenda is no longer running marathons. She uses an assistive device when she walks. Her symptoms are visible. Back when she saw that first neurologist, I ask, what part of her identity did she think doctors might be most prejudiced about? Her young age? Her gender? Her race?

"When my disability wasn't as pronounced," she says, "I worried that I wouldn't be taken as seriously because I am a Latina woman." And now that her disability from the neurological disease is much more obvious to outsiders, she notices a big difference when someone else is with her.

"I know that my white husband will get more done than a Latina woman," she says, referring to his receiving more attention or respect—and hence, action—from staff. He comes with her to almost every appointment.

I mention to Brenda that I've had some funny and not-so-funny moments along these lines. As a white Jewish woman, I don't have to worry much about racism. But doctors sometimes seem to dismiss me as a woman, a young woman. So a few years ago, I asked Simon, who was always offering to accompany me if I wanted him to, to meet me at a doctor's appointment. A man, I figured, and a man who looks a bit older than I do, might help. But, Simon and I joked, given that he's a black man, if the doctor ended up being more racist than misogynistic, the effort would be no good. Only if the doctor cared more about a man in the room might this kind of socially conferred authority, regardless of race, help. Otherwise, the reality is that his presence, depending on the doctor, could hurt.

What a ridiculous calculation to try to make, I say to Brenda. To hope for a doctor who's more sexist than racist? It sounds like a joke. But Brenda agrees that it's real.

And my desire to bring Simon to the doctor, I realize, is probably rooted in the time a trusted doctor sexually harassed me. No one else, regardless of gender or race, was in the room for that.

———

Bias against young women in the medical arena comes up in a few major ways. It can happen at the doctor's office or hospital, where we're seeking health care, with doctors not believing us. There's a millennia-long history of it. It can also happen in more directly violent ways: sexual harassment and assault by medical staff. And then, beyond the patient-doctor interaction, bias happens all the time in ways we don't see: health research that overlooks young women, women of color, and women in general. For young women going to various physicians and specialists, all these forces can be at play. Miriam, the assistant principal of an El Paso high school, ended up with stage 3 cancer. The outcome might have been different had her doctor listened to her earlier. When she found a lump in her breast, she told her doctor. She got an ultrasound. The doctor said it was fine. Then she went back to the doctor when she found another lump. Still fine, the doctor said. Maybe she should take antibiotics, in case it's an infection.

Then, her symptoms got worse: extreme pain that penetrated back to her shoulder blade; blood in her bra. The doctor kept saying it might be something more minor, not cancer, and that she was fine.

Something in Miriam told her that this wasn't the case, she says, but as a young woman, she felt too intimidated to contradict a physician who had authority and knowledge over her.

"How do you go against a doctor who has a PhD or a medical license or whatever," she says, "smarter than you or more experienced than you, who's older than you, who you have to trust—how do I tell them they're wrong?" When she looks back at how powerless she felt and what allowed her doctor to ignore her symptoms, Miriam says, "I don't think it's just my culture, because I'm Hispanic, but I think it's because I was young and because I was timid."

The fourth time Miriam saw her doctor and discussed the blood in her bra, the doctor had already given her two ultrasounds.

"Her words were, 'I don't know what else you want me to do.' And something inside of me got really mad," Miriam says, "and I just lost it. . . . What do you mean, what else you want me to do? There must be another test."

Finally, the doctor said she could give Miriam an MRI.

But even with this next step suddenly materializing, Miriam wasn't informed. She didn't know that not every place does breast MRIs or that you have to do it within a few days of your period. She had to learn all these things for the first time, she says, in an uphill battle to get the test she needed. It was around the end of December, and many medical facilities were closed. After the new year, she went to a clinic for breast care, where the staff members said they couldn't see her till April.

That was it. Miriam, who was presenting with bloody discharge and extreme pain, cried when she heard there were no spots open for months. The office staff saw her reaction and said they could squeeze her in sooner between other appointments.

The next obstacle: Miriam's insurance didn't want to pay for the MRI she'd just fought for. And her insurance refused to pay for a mammogram, too, presumably because she was under forty.

"If a woman encounters all of those obstacles, at some point we're going to give up," Miriam says. "I don't think I'd be here if I had given up."

We can't really trust in the medical system to advocate for us or take care of us, she adds. We have to know what our rights are and just keep pushing for care.

"I do think that's a problem and I do think a lot of it has to do with being young and not knowing better," she says.

"I didn't know that I could leave . . . and find another doctor and that my insurance would cover it." She says she didn't know that you don't have to go to the imaging lab the doctor writes down or that a patient can ask for a copy of her records every time she goes to the doctor, or that her doctor can vouch for her if the insurance company at first refuses to cover a necessary test.

Finally, Miriam advocated more for herself and got more testing. A different doctor did a biopsy, and after restless days waiting for the results, Miriam was back at his office, her husband in tow. She sat at the edge of the exam table, her feet dangling, waiting.

"He walks in and he's just real matter-of-fact," she says of the doctor. "'Oh yeah, you do have cancer.'"

Miriam says, "My brain and my mouth and my heart, they were not communicating with each other. I felt sick. I felt like someone had put their hand down my throat and pulled my heart out."

The doctor just kept going. "I need you to schedule an appointment," he told Miriam. "You're gonna come back in two or three weeks, and I'll see you then."

Despite feeling out of her body, Miriam managed to ask what would happen at that next appointment.

"Well, you're gonna tell me if you want a single or double mastectomy," the doctor said. No explanation. At that point, Miriam only knew the word *mastectomy* from having done research. Otherwise, she would have had no idea what it even referred to. The doctor made no move to explain it.

She asked the doctor if that was it. He said yes. Miriam's husband asked if this would affect her ability to have children. Yes, the doctor said. He said nothing else.

Miriam broke down in tears. Her husband hugged her. The doctor's phone rang, and he was gone.

"It was ugly the way he did it," Miriam tells me. "It's like *ahhhh*, okay, *boom*, here you go." During that appointment, the physician didn't tell Miriam what stage cancer she had or even that there were different types of breast cancer. She didn't find that out until later, when she went to another doctor.

After the doctor left, Miriam was still in tears. A nurse handed her a tissue and told her she could stay in the room as long as she needed. Miriam can't remember the doctor's face, but she remembers the nurse whose kindness made her feel safe for a moment.

But Miriam, like several other women I've interviewed, says she does have empathy for doctors, even ones who seem callous or cruel in these moments. Maybe, she says, they're protecting themselves and have become desensitized to the human aspect of practicing medicine. A kind of defense mechanism to get through seeing patients who might not live much longer.

More recently, a young woman, under forty, came to Miriam. She'd been having unusual symptoms and was afraid it was breast cancer. When she told Miriam the name of the doctor she'd been going to, it was the same one who had denied that anything was wrong with Miriam over the course of four appointments and increasingly alarming symptoms. Miriam realized that the same thing was happening again: the same doctor was seeing a patient who was under forty and presenting with symptoms similar to Miriam's and telling her, as she'd told Miriam, that she was fine.

Miriam was mad. She told the young woman to stop seeing that doctor and go to someone else. She wanted to know how to stop this same pattern from happening. She considered bringing a suit against the doctor. But, she learned, the statute of limitations where she lives begins the moment symptoms begin, not when a patient finally gets a diagnosis, and lasts just two years. As she was going through treatment for her cancer, the window of time was closing. The attorney she consulted said that it would be a hard case for him, and costly. He said Miriam could also make a complaint to the Texas medical board, but she didn't have the energy. She had to get through the chemo.

At the very least, Miriam says, she'd like to sit down with the doctor who kept telling her she was fine and who did the same to the other young woman Miriam met. Miriam wants to tell the doctor that she ended up having stage 3 cancer, rather than stage 1, after all that time waiting for testing. To show the doctor the real cost of not taking a patient seriously.

Miriam shares another moment she had with a physician—this episode perhaps more hopeful. When, in the middle of her cancer treatment, Miriam wasn't feeling well, she went to an urgent-care clinic. There she saw a doctor, a woman about her age, and told her story: the many missed chances for diagnosis, the way the first doctor had ignored the urgency of her symptoms.

And then, the urgent-care doctor started to cry.

Miriam wondered if it was because of something personal. "Do you know someone who has cancer?" she asked.

"No," the physician said, "it's not that." Then she made a confession: "I would have done everything the same as that doctor. I would have gone with the ultrasound results. I would have thought you looked healthy."

Miriam told the doctor that there must be a reason they had had this conversation. "Please remember my story, and treat each of your patients as individuals, and listen to them—they know their bodies best," she said.

And the doctor hugged her.

———

I take the train to Columbia University to meet with Alondra Nelson, the university's dean of social science and the author of several books on medicine and race, including *The Social Life of DNA: Race, Reparations, and Reconciliation After the Genome* and *Body and Soul: The Black Panther Party and the Fight Against Medical Discrimination.* As we sit at a table in her office, a room within a famous building built in the Roman style and topped by a dome, I ask her a question that I admit may sound odd. Of the many terrible types of discrimination in medicine that persist today, could she choose one that's been documented with data and seems to rise above the rest in its awfulness? It seems silly, in a way, to try to narrow down all these manifestations of oppression, but I'm curious what stands out to her.

"There have been some recent studies around pain—and stigma, and criminalization, and the sort of unholy alliance of those three things," she says. Persons of color, she says, are probably disproportionately not believed by doctors when they say they are in pain. "They're always considered unreliable narrators. And not only unreliable narrators, but criminals, or addicts, or people who are seeking drugs rather than seeking healing or seeking alleviation of pain."

One 2016 study, by Kelly Hoffman, a postdoctoral fellow at Northwestern University, and her colleagues, sought to understand past findings that doctors ignore black patients' pain more than they do white patients'. It found that "a substantial number of white laypeople and medical students and [medical] residents hold false beliefs about biological differences between blacks and whites"—false ideas such as one race having more nerve endings than the other, or thicker skin, or stronger immune systems.[2] A staggering half of those surveyed believed at least one of these ideas, the study found. And those who had these false conceptions had a racial bias in how they perceived black patients' pain or prescribed treatment. They didn't take black patients' pain seriously.

There is a long history of racist and classist stereotypes when it comes to women's bodies. As Barbara Ehrenreich and Deirdre English write in *Complaints & Disorders: The Sexual Politics of Sickness*, in the late nineteenth and early twentieth centuries, "affluent women were seen as inherently sick, too weak and delicate for anything but the mildest pastimes, while working-class women were believed to be inherently healthy and robust."[3] These harmful stereotypes, which, among other problems, led to disparities in health-care access, served to reinforce social divides—and to bolster capitalism. People in the leisure class could go on with their light activities and their rest, but, as Ehrenreich and English write, "*someone* had to be well enough to do the work." Conveniently, as one doctor at the time wrote, the stereotypical black woman "who toils beside her husband in the fields of the south" or "who washes, and scrubs and toils in our homes at the north, enjoy for the most part good health, with comparative immunity from uterine disease."[4] This attitude, Ehrenreich and English find, is representative of the thinking at the time. (And I'd say the way the doctor writes "our homes" gives his motives away even more plainly.)

This type of thinking about bodies, race, and pain dates back much further, too, to one of the justifications white people used for slavery in the United States. Hoffman and her coauthors acknowledge this ill-intentioned argument. "Beliefs that blacks and whites are fundamentally and biologically different have been prevalent in various forms for centuries," they write. "In the United States, these beliefs were championed by scientists, physicians, and slave owners alike to justify slavery and the inhumane treatment of black men and women in medical research."[5] But these false ideas have not yet gone away.

While stereotypes about race and class undoubtedly affect how health practitioners view a person's capacity for pain, some false beliefs affect women more broadly, regardless of background. A study from 2001 suggests that health-care providers take women's pain less seriously; dismiss women's pain as "emotional," "psychogenic," and "not real" more often than they do men's pain; and even assume that women are not in pain if they're physically attractive.[6] Perhaps these findings are not so surprising to those of us who've heard "But you look great!" in response to "My joints hurt."

Racism, sexism, and misogyny, Nelson says, are in the room with the patient and the doctor right from the start of the medical encounter. These types of bias, or bigotry, enter the space "before anybody's even uttered a word or said anything about potential disease or what might be the potential solution to what people are feeling," she says. "And so that means . . . folks of color, poor folks, are never given the benefit of the doubt." Doctors often assume "that a claim about pain always has an ulterior motive."

What's especially challenging, Nelson says, is that human suffering, human vulnerability, is usually what we turn to when we want to find the universal thread that unites human beings. As she puts it, "that's been the thing that we can say: 'We eat different food, and we have different languages, and we worship different gods, but we're all humans and we all have this vulnerability.' When that very vulnerability, and that very sense of suffering, is put in question, it makes it very difficult, I think, for people to get well."

A woman named Samira writes that she's a "twenty-nine-year-old woman of color/femmedrogynous person of color" who came out as queer when she was thirteen, though she didn't pursue queer relationships until she moved to New York at twenty-four.

"I was diagnosed with posttraumatic stress disorder at eighteen," she tells me. "At twenty-two, I was diagnosed with polycystic ovarian syndrome. When I was twenty-four, my mental health diagnosis shifted to complex posttraumatic stress disorder. When I was twenty-six, hypothyroidism. When I was twenty-eight, severe IBS [irritable bowel syndrome]. And as of a month ago, [I] was just put on metformin for insulin-resistance issues linked to my PCOS [polycystic ovarian syndrome]."

Despite this combination of serious—and diagnosed—health issues, Samira cannot get doctors to listen.

"I live with chronic pain," she writes, "but am refused any form of reprieve from my practitioners. They don't see the pain, exhaustion, anxiety, or depression that have become a part of my conditions as enough reason to provide me with medication to help. I try to do acupuncture when I can, I go to therapy two times a week." Still, she says, "I've dealt with homophobia and misdiagnosis"—and, it seems, the common belief that her pain isn't worth treating or even real.

The history of ignoring or disbelieving women's pain is centuries old. The problem is so vast that it's almost too unwieldy, too pervasive throughout history, to summarize briefly.

Someone recommends a TED talk to me. The speaker is Jennifer Brea, a former PhD candidate who came down with a fever of 104.7.[7] "After the fever broke," Brea says, "for three weeks I was so dizzy, I couldn't leave my house. I would walk straight into door frames. I had to hug the walls just to make it to the bathroom." Soon she started to get an array of infections, too. Doctors said it was nothing. Then, she says, neurological symptoms began. She couldn't draw the right side of a circle anymore. Sometimes, she couldn't move.

Conversion disorder, the neurologist told her. Also known as hysteria. Maybe a trauma that she'd never dealt with was causing her pain—pain that was in her head.

After that false diagnosis, she walked two miles home, pushing herself to understand how the excruciating zaps of pain going through her were something her body was fabricating. The walk wreaked havoc on her. She couldn't move, she couldn't think. She has, she says, never been the same since.

Myalgic encephalomyelitis, it turns out, was what she had. Not some imaginary syndrome, as might be asserted by misogynistic doctors. This disease, formerly known as chronic fatigue syndrome, is often medically overlooked and, for many people, is extremely grave.

"The ignorance surrounding my disease has been a choice," she says. "A choice made by the institutions that were supposed to protect us." And myalgic encephalomyelitis, she reports, "affects women at two to three times the rate of men. This issue is much bigger than just my disease. When I first got sick, old friends were reaching out to me. And I soon found myself part of a cohort of women in their late twenties whose bodies were falling apart. What was striking was just how much trouble we were having being taken seriously."

Brea recalls "one woman with scleroderma, an autoimmune connective-tissue disease, who was told for years that it was all in her head." Between the time that woman first started experiencing symptoms to when she finally was diagnosed properly, Brea says, "her esophagus was so thoroughly damaged, she will never be able to eat again."

But it's not just with autoimmune issues, this medical disbelief. This prejudice affects the treatment of all types of diseases a woman might have. Brea talks about a woman with symptoms "who for years was told that it was just early menopause." The symptoms turned out to be the result of ovarian cancer. And then there's the friend from college, she says, who for years was misdiagnosed with anxiety.

It was, in fact, a brain tumor.


Danielle is a gynecological oncology surgeon who specializes in women's cancers. She herself has the BRCA gene mutation—a mutation that increases the risk of breast cancer—so she decided to have a double mastectomy for preventive reasons. I speak with her awhile before the surgery, and then after. The operation went relatively well, she tells me afterward, aside from some minor complications. But she did learn a bit about what her patients are going through.

"I don't think being a doctor has made me a better patient," she says. "I think being a patient has made me a better doctor." She had many fears leading up to her surgery: Will it go okay? Will she be okay? Will the surgeon do the reconstruction she wanted that day, or will she wake up and learn that it was too complicated and that she has to wait several months before she can look like herself again? Now, she says, she has a little more empathy for the women she's about to perform surgery on. And the main complication she did experience, though not severe, has shifted the way she does and doesn't pay attention to her patients' symptoms and pain.

"The day after my surgery," she says, "I was having trouble moving my left arm. And everyone was like, 'Oh yeah, that's your nondominant arm, so that's not totally surprising.' And I was like, okay, seems like a really legitimate answer." But Danielle knew that she should be able to move both arms ninety degrees. She could do so with her right arm. With her left, she could still only lift it just forty-five degrees. Doctors kept saying the same thing: "Your right arm is just stronger." She listened to her doctors.

Then, about a month into her recovery, she was in the shower. For weeks she had just let the soapy water run over the surgical area, never touching it directly. Finally, this time, she did.

"And I felt this huge piece of scar tissue holding my left arm down," she says. "Essentially, it felt like a violin string between my upper and lower—right in my armpit—holding my left arm down."

She started googling. *Mastectomy string. Mastectomy chord. Mastectomy armpit*—all the keywords she thought would help her diagnose it. Because she's a doctor, she says, she was able to take what she found online and look through the medical library, to read the literature for herself. She figured it out.

So she called one of her doctors. "'I have chording syndrome,'" she told the doctor. "'That's why I can't move my left arm.' And suddenly they took me seriously, and they were like, 'You have to go to physical therapy immediately.'"

Had she not been a doctor herself, Danielle says, she would have probably continued to describe it in lay terms—"there's this weird thing in my armpit"—and it would have probably taken days for her to see anyone about it. Because she switched to medical language, because she was an insider, her doctor did a complete turnaround and not only listened to her, but also called ahead to her physical therapist for her.

That was the privilege of being a doctor, she says.

"You know those studies about doctors not listening to women's pain?" I ask.

"*I'm* one of those doctors a lot of the time, unfortunately," Danielle says.

At this point, I make some kind of surprised sound. She herself does this to patients? But she continues.

"That's actually one of the reasons that I went into cancer," she says. "Because I can't—I have trouble dealing with vague things that I can't [diagnose]. Just my personality." Although she entered medical school with the goal of becoming a primary care doctor, she soon found that she had no patience for confusing symptoms, chronic pain. She realized she works better when the situation is cut-and-dried: cancer or no cancer. Not all the murky in-between.

"I think that's really great," I say, "that you're meta-cognizant of it and know your personality wouldn't work with those situations and patients. But some people with your personality do seem to become those types of doctors."

"That's terrible!" she says. She knows that these doctors' incompatible choices aren't good for patients and adds, "I have a lot of friends who are pelvic pain specialists. . . . They listen. They talk to patients about it." Danielle admires her friends who practice this type of medicine, in which the cause of pain is not as easy to track down as, say, the tumors that she deals with as a surgeon. "You are sooo great," she tells them. "I don't have the patience for that."

"And so," she says, "I understand what my doctors were doing." Danielle impersonates herself complaining about her limited range of motion: "I can't move my left aaaaarm," she jokes, giving me a caricature of herself as an annoying patient. "They didn't do a physical exam," she says, and they should have. They would have found the issue sooner, and she would have healed faster, with more range of motion, and not had to go to physical therapy three times a week, more than the average patient who has had a mastectomy.

"I just found that entire thing incredibly frustrating," she says. Because her doctors didn't listen to her complaints and, as she puts it, basically said she was being silly, her complication from the surgery got worse. "And so now," she says, "I take patients' concerns a little more seriously. I think nine out of ten times, I probably don't need to, and it's just the normal recovery process and there's nothing to worry about. But I think of that *one* patient—you know?"

———

Gwyneth Ferguson Matthews, writing in *Voices from the Shadows* in 1983, recalls the different (misogynistic) ways doctors treated her as a woman with a visible disability. One doctor, she says, discouraged her from having kids, even though she could conceive, because he didn't think she could handle them afterward from her wheelchair. Still, he was kinder than another physician Matthews saw. This one, Dr. Landers, "showed me just how rotten doctors' attitudes vis-à-vis their disabled patients can be, particularly regarding sex and childbearing."[8] Matthews came to him after she'd had a miscarriage. His response was that she shouldn't have children, period.

"By the time they'd be five or six," he told Matthews, "you'd have them doing so much fetching and carrying they'd hate you, and by the time they reached their teens, you'd have no social values to pass on to them."

Matthews recalls being stunned, in disbelief that a physician would say something like this.

"Wait a minute," she said to the doctor. "I have a normal marriage, and my husband and I are hardly social outcasts. We go everywhere and do everything other couples do. I may be a paraplegic, but you're treating me like a cripple!"

The distinction between a person with a disability and the slur Matthews referred to seemed to escape the doctor, who, Matthews writes, "continued as if I hadn't spoken." What he said next was unsolicited and even more out of line.

"If your husband ever tires of a paraplegic wife," he told Matthews—seemingly apropos of nothing—"you must be understanding." And then: "You should encourage him to seek company elsewhere; help him find a nice mistress."

While that may sound like an outrageous example, there are still doctors who make their patients feel erased. A woman named Yukiko experienced it recently.

"For a long time," she tells me, "I did not make space to think about or grieve [over] all that being chronically ill has meant in my life." We're typing to each other over G-chat before she has an appointment. It's easier with her schedule.

Yukiko has type 1 diabetes, though she writes, "I am type 1 diabetic." Her phrasing makes me think about the push for people-first language that some advocate, the shift from "I am *a* diabetic," for instance, to "I am a *person with* diabetes." Yukiko, who's thirty-two, tells me she identifies as a queer, mixed-race, Japanese American, and Jewish clinical social worker–psychotherapist. Throughout our conversation, it's apparent that she thinks a lot about identity. So I wonder if she is simply used to the phrasing she uses or if she actively identifies that way, choosing to make diabetes a part of herself with her wording. Different women I've met have used various terms and ways of framing things. Several have shared their thoughts on whether they identify as someone disabled, someone *with* a disability, or someone with health issues.

Victoria Rodriguez-Roldan, of the National LGBTQ Task Force, for instance, makes a point of calling her bipolar disorder a disability, not a health issue. She says that people-first language can be great if a person with a disability chooses to use it, but that it can also come from a not-so-great place. Using language that distances people from their disability, she says, can stem from a way of thinking that "disability is so horrible that I don't want to be identified with it." And, she adds, "many people feel that their disability is an integral part of themselves," especially in the autistic and Deaf communities, but also among plenty of other people with disabilities. Each person should be able to decide, she says, whether they want to say, "I have diabetes" or "I am a diabetic," "I am disabled" or "I have a disability."

When I tell Rodriguez-Roldan that I don't think of myself as someone either disabled *or* with a disability, since I just have "a bunch of weird serious health issues," she gets at what a few other women I'd met have said: Why not? She uses the term *mental health disability* for herself, or *psychiatric disability*, as opposed to *mental health issue*. And she does so purposefully. As a lawyer, she's aware of how language helps legitimize what's covered by the Americans with Disabilities Act. She thinks that people with serious health issues that affect their day-to-day lives shouldn't have a hierarchy of what's "disabled enough" to count—nor should only certain types of bodies represent the wide array of bodies that make up humanity.

"The people who get to be at the press conference, the people who get to do the lobbying, the people who get to be in the picture on the website," she says, are usually "the people with the 'sexy' disability. There will probably be a person in a wheelchair, maybe with a cane if blind. White, photogenic, often male, almost invariably cis and straight, maybe a token gay person. They will often exclude the person with the developmental disability, the person with the mental health disability, the person who is not 'pretty,' so to speak, or whose physical disability is not what we consider photogenic." And, Rodriguez-Roldan says, if you've got a long list of health issues that affect you every day (as I do), that seems like living with disability.

Back with Yukiko. Before I can ask about her choice of words, she continues. "Physically, I am 'able-bodied' to a large extent, but diabetes is debilitating physically," she types. And, she adds, reading my mind about this very subject, "diabetes was added to the ADA [Americans with Disabilities Act] list of disabilities, which I think is a good thing." She says that she is not always "able-bodied," and that when it comes to diabetes, "the mental impact is huge." The disease, she explains, is minute-to-minute. In her case, it means giving herself at least five injections a day and testing her blood sugar levels at least ten times a day.

"Those are the interventions," she says. "But the bigger part is just a constant attention to and dealing with fluctuating glucose levels, with lows leading to dizziness, exhaustion, confusion, fear, anxiety, et cetera." High levels, she says, involve thirst, migraines and other headaches, and fear about all the long-term issues she knows high levels can lead to: heart attack, stroke, blindness, amputations.

When it comes to health care, she says, "I usually seek care from doctors of color to avoid racist interactions." Likewise, she seeks female doctors, to try to avoid misogyny. Still, "the queer stuff can be hard. I wish all my doctors were queer."

Indeed, Yukiko and her partner ran up against some upsetting moments at the doctor's office a few years ago. They wanted children, and Yukiko was the one who would get pregnant.

Yukiko worked for years, she says, to get her blood levels safe enough to conceive. She had always wanted to prove that her body, which she says often feels broken, could carry a pregnancy and give birth. Additionally, her partner is gender nonconforming and didn't feel inclined to become pregnant: it would have set off gender dysphoria for her. She would have done it if it were a last resort, Yukiko says, but when they went together to see various obstetricians about how to proceed, they made it quite clear that Yukiko would be the one to carry. Several doctors, however, didn't listen, in ways that felt traumatizing.

"The biggest asshole I met," Yukiko writes, "was a team of them: [a] high-risk obstetrics practice who did that whole . . . reductive story thing where they were like 'the cool thing about you two being lesbians . . . ' (we don't ID as lesbians) 'is that you have TWO UTERUSES!'"

One of doctors on the team, a woman who, Yukiko believes, identifies herself as a sort of "capital-L lesbian" (i.e., someone who doesn't see the more nuanced versions of queer identity), was especially hurtful. Despite Yukiko's having come in as the patient who would be getting pregnant, the doctor pointed at Yukiko's partner and said, "She can and should obviously be the pregnant one!"

In an instant, Yukiko says, she negated Yukiko's own longing to carry a child, which the couple had been abundantly straightforward about, as well as her partner's complete lack of interest in becoming pregnant. Instead of professionally discussing any concerns, the doctor disregarded that the couple was already extremely informed about how diabetes complicated things and that Yukiko had been working to get her body in the best possible place for pregnancy. That the doctor was herself a lesbian didn't help—and maybe even hurt.

"It was really bad," Yukiko tells me, "and also unfortunate because they were the first practice we interviewed. So it started us out feeling defeated, which was hard to overcome."

As a therapist, Yukiko sees this resigned reaction in many of her clients, too. They have a bad experience or two with a clinician who is, as Yukiko puts it, "mis-attuned to their experience of their health, gender, sexual orientation, or all three," and so they stop seeking the care they need.

For Yukiko and her own partner, it wasn't just this first doctor who acted like this. "We got that a lot," she says, "like telling us who we are, and what our experience is, and what we 'should' do based on it." All these experiences felt horrible. And it took a while to find a doctor who listened.

"I do feel very lucky that we found a high-risk ob[stetrician] who was so supportive of our identities and relationship," she says. In the end, Yukiko and her partner had a midwife come to their house and help with intrauterine insemination. By the time we spoke, their son was seventeen months old.

———

I ask Jayde about doctors—Jayde, the thirty-one-year-old who is trying to cope with polyps in her stomach and a tumor in her brain. I ask if she thinks physicians interact with her a certain way because she's young, or a woman, or a woman of color. I'm not prepared for the intensity of her stories.

"Yeah, I had that," she says. "When I was first diagnosed, the doctor was—well, he actually made me cry. The staff was actually afraid to touch me, 'cause they thought they were gonna catch something. So they told my grandmother what to do to help me, 'cause I was in so much pain, and I had to have some ointment put on my skin."

This happened after she'd had her colon removed. It is still a difficult surgery today, but when Jayde had the surgery, it was newer to medicine and therefore not something even the surgeon was used to.

After that type of surgery, she says, "it's kind of gross. You have to go [to the bathroom] a lot. So your skin, it wears down. The doctor didn't know what to do. So my doctor came up with treating me like a baby, in a way." The medical staff on her floor didn't understand what was going on with her skin, and they thought it was contagious. They wouldn't touch her. Jayde was only sixteen.

She was in a lot of pain. But doctors also yelled at her a lot, she remembers. Luckily, her grandmother never left her side.

"I remember lying there [thinking], 'If you wouldn't touch me, I wonder how you treat people with AIDS in this hospital.' And I'm dealing with cancer," she says.

But, Jayde goes on to explain, something more disturbing happened to her.

"After I had the colon surgery, my doctor sent me to have this special X-ray, and I remember going down there to the room and I remember this was when I was just trying to learn to stand back up on my two feet. . . . I was cut wide open, so you know my stomach, everything, it hurts. This doctor wanted me to bend over. And I was trying to tell him I couldn't."

Jayde said that it hurt too much. "He got angry with me," she remembers. "And when I say he got angry, he got *physical* with me. I'm a teenager, and my grandmother is outside. Because it's an X-ray room, she couldn't be in the room with me. She's outside the door, and you know those doors are really thick? So I don't think she could really hear me. He got so angry with me, he pushed me over." Then he lifted her up, took the tube out of her nose, and stuck it back in. "He's literally physically shoving me," she says.

"It's not a regular X-ray machine," she says. "I forget what kind of machine it is, but you stand up, and sometimes you drink stuff and they take pictures. But because I have the tube in my nose, I can't drink stuff, and he's pulling stuff out, and he's literally getting physical with me, and I'm a child, and he takes me by my neck, and he starts shoving me, almost, like, my head could touch my toes."

Here was a kid, spending a month in the ICU. Instead of a regular life at school, she'd just had her colon cut out and was in terrible pain. And a medical professional was assaulting her. I think about not only the findings that doctors disbelieve women and black patients about pain, but also about the research on how Americans view black children as threatening adults.[9] The same type of thinking behind cops who see black teens and choose to kill them.

Jayde continues. "One of his staff members came in after . . . and physically grabbed him by the collar and pulled him off of me. And they started tussling. And that's when my grandmother heard and bum-rushed in, and she sees me on the floor crying and she's like, 'What did he do?' And the staff member tried to explain to her."

Ever since then, Jayde says, if she needs to go into an X-ray room, she has to have somebody with her. She also stopped going to the hospital where it happened. Too scary.

The man who assaulted her physically wasn't just pushing her and screaming at her, she tells me, as if that weren't enough. She cleans up the man's words when she says them to me, but the sharpness is still there.

"He was like, 'You lazy m-f-ing patients come in here,' and I was like, 'Oh my gosh.' I was like, 'This is besides having bad bed manner.'"

At this point, listening to Jayde's excruciating experience, I'm ticking off the stereotypes this guy at the hospital has thrown at her. First, despite her being a teenager who had just undergone traumatic surgery and would never have a colon or a regular digestive system again, despite her having spent a month in intensive care and barely being able to walk on her own, he ignored her when she said she was in pain—just as research has shown happens with both women and black patients.

The man also called her lazy—a racist remark.

Another health-care worker, a doctor, lobbed a racial stereotype at Jayde, too. He accused Jayde's grandmother of trying to make

Jayde a drug addict. Since her pain didn't seem real to this physician, he went for the idea that the meds she needed were for a substance-abuse problem, rather than the searing pain a girl would be likely to experience after her intestines had been ripped apart.

"I should be able to come into the doctor and trust that when I'm sitting across the table from my doctor, they should listen to me," she says. "I shouldn't come in here and get chills just being in this room. They take something extremely important away from you. And it's very, very hard to get it back."

You're already putting your life in someone's hands, Jayde says. "You're already saying, 'Here's my life—it's up to you to help me.' So when someone takes that and says, 'Now I'm gonna control you,' it's very hard for you to trust somebody else."

Jayde describes another moment that made her feel unwelcome and unsafe around doctors, despite her constant need to rely on them to stay alive.

"This was the anesthesiologist as he was putting me to sleep," she says. "He was literally putting the needle in my arm and putting me to sleep—and he told me, 'You must not give a crap about yourself.' And I was like, 'What are you talking about?' And it was at the time where I had gained a lot of weight. And suddenly—I didn't gain the weight by choice. I gained weight because my thyroid was totally out of whack at the time. They had just found out the best dosage for my thyroid medicine, and I'd already lost forty pounds. . . . But I guess he had a problem finding . . . a vein to put an IV in my arm, and he was like, 'You must not care about yourself.'"

Jayde asked why he would say that. "Because you're obese," he said, "and I don't understand why somebody like you who's this sick would get carried away like this. Why would you sit here and get fat."

Jayde couldn't say much, as the anesthesia kicked in. The last thing she heard as her surgery began was a doctor telling her she was fat.


Jayde's experience might sound shocking. But because of the power dynamics involved, because patients still need medical treatment and are often still at the mercy of those who harm them, this kind of experience is also probably underreported: emotional and physical, as well as sexual, abuse.

In 2016, *Gothamist* reported on a doctor at a large, well-known institution in Manhattan, and one where I happened to go for cancer surgery and follow-up visits. He had repeatedly sexually assaulted his patients.[10] The *Gothamist* piece described the particulars:

> Dr. David Newman turned himself in to Special Victims Unit detectives yesterday after a young female patient, 29, said he sexually assaulted her when she went to Mount Sinai Hospital for shoulder pain. She was first given pills and morphine from a nurse, but when Newman checked on her, he allegedly gave her more morphine, even though the patient said she had been given a dose. . . . While she went in and out of consciousness, he fondled her breasts, and ejaculated on her face. The patient then saved the blanket Newman allegedly used to wipe semen from her face as well as a hospital gown that she used to wipe remaining ejaculate. He is charged with sexual abuse and forcible touching.

Once that story came out, another woman came forward with a similar story.

———

Alondra Nelson puts it this way: historically, the places where marginalized populations go for access to health care have often felt unsafe or have overlooked whole groups of people, "oscillating between neglect and abuse."

As a young white woman, I have never been physically assaulted in a hospital or called names. Nothing that medical professionals have done to me has come anywhere close. And yet, there's that typical line of thought—the insidious idea that often prevents women from reporting traumatic or illegal incidents: *It wasn't that bad. Other women have had it worse.*

When it comes to rape, sexual assault, sexual harassment, catcalling, and other street harassment—all of which, some have pointed out, are on the same continuum—this thinking is quite common.[11]

Women often minimize what has happened to them, for a number of complex reasons related to internalized misogyny, feeling powerless or scared, or not wanting to take up space or accuse someone of something that "wasn't that bad." I've heard countless women say to me, "Well, he didn't touch me; he only said this awful thing," or, "Since it wasn't 'full' rape, I didn't think it was worth reporting." Or the other reason: "I didn't know if anyone would believe me."

I've often marveled at the lengths my peers have gone to in minimizing what has happened to them. When they downplay what someone said or did because it wasn't as awful as other stories they've heard, I've often thought, "No! Resist!" Then I realized that I've done the same downplaying.

My pharmacist seemed like a relatively thoughtful guy. I went to his independent store because I have to take three pills just to keep going every day, even though I used to be someone who eschewed medicine. I figured I could at least support a local business instead of a big drugstore chain. But every time I visited the store, the pharmacist would say, "Miiiiiissssssss Hirsch, what a beauuuutiful smile," or, "You're so *pretty*, Miss Hirsch, you make me sing." The first time, I chalked it up to his being in a good mood—he had a line of customers waiting for their prescriptions and the radio tuned to Motown hits. But then it kept happening, every month. Not a big deal, I thought, till I realized I was steeling my shoulders when I walked in and trying to avoid eye contact with him. I was dreading the day each month when I'd smile weakly back at his perhaps well-meaning but unwanted harassment.

For a long time, I wouldn't have dared call it that word, harassment. It was casual and innocent, I thought. He was a friendly guy, wasn't he? Then I realized that not only was I steeling my shoulders before entering his store—I was also bracing myself on other days that I happened to walk down that block. I would see the sign for his pharmacy, sometimes glimpse him through the jingling glass door, and notice that all my muscles would lock together in knots.

It felt like such a stupid reason to switch pharmacies, though, given that he had all my information on file and I had a complicated insurance policy. But when, a few months later, I saw that a new independent pharmacy had opened a few blocks away, I went in to the new place to ask about switching my prescriptions over. When the new pharmacist asked where I'd be switching from, I felt guilty, as if he'd somehow figure out why I was leaving the old place. But I switched nevertheless.

The new pharmacist was great. He never commented on my looks or how my body made him feel. What a low bar I was holding him to: he was "great" because he didn't harass me.

There was another incident I'd been having trouble categorizing or ranking, when in fact, any unethical or illegal behavior toward patients ranks as intolerable. But compared with my pharmacist interaction, this incident was worse, even as I continue to fight the habit of saying, "Oh, but compared with what has happened to other people, it's not *that* bad." (I do push against this impulse, knowing that when we agree to diminish ourselves and our experiences of misogyny, it helps keep the patriarchy well-oiled.) And unlike with the pharmacist whom I could get away from, this has continued to affect my access to vital health care.

I met the doctor just a few weeks after the anaphylaxis episodes that had nearly killed me. I was still shaky whenever I left my home. An allergist in Manhattan had sent me to him because, she said, after lots of testing, she thought my condition was beyond her specialty. A doctor whose last name was Valla, she'd said, was the only person within hundreds of miles of the city who knew about the syndrome she thought I had. So although we were in a major urban center, one of the biggest in the world, I'd have to take a regional rail for two hours, then a commuter bus for another hour, and visit Valla in the remote suburb where he practiced.

During my first appointment, Valla was warm. His eyes widened as I told him what had happened in New York and in India. "I'm not sure how you're alive," he said, in a whisper reminiscent of when my coworker Michael compared me to a ghost. The doctor said the symptoms did sound like what he specialized in: a rare condition called idiopathic anaphylaxis, sometimes named mast-cell activation syndrome. A special urine test he ordered confirmed the diagnosis. He told me that the condition was dangerous, but that he had about eight other patients with idiopathic anaphylaxis and he could help guide me through it and manage my medicine. And so, despite trembling every time I remembered what had happened, how my body was fine one minute and throwing me into asphyxiation the next, each time I met with Valla, I felt safe.

One day, after my three-hour trip, I sat in Valla's exam room, asking him about a strange symptom I'd been having. Out of nowhere, a lascivious smirk spread across his face. His eyes changed.

"You're lucky you're cute," he said, his voice slow, purposeful, suddenly sexual. "Or I might not answer all your questions."

He raised his eyebrows. I froze. I looked at this doctor, who'd made me feel less scared about my body over the past few years. Now, he was the one who scared me. I looked to the door to see if we were locked into the room together. It was slightly ajar. For the rest of the appointment, my brain was on autopilot.

I can't come back here, I thought when I got out. I didn't want to know what other line he might have crossed if the door to the room had been closed. But when I tried to find another doctor who had experience with my syndrome, I found no one. There was a reason the first allergist had sent me to the remote town. Valla was the only one who could help. Even the urine test he had ordered every year to monitor my levels was impossible to find at another doctor's office. Because of the mayhem that is our country's insurance system, the simple test was allowed in some places, but not New York. Valla had a special double license in another state that allowed him to prescribe it. I was dependent on his office.

So the next year, I weighed the risks. I decided to go to him again, since nobody else had his specialty, even if it meant he might do something worse. Knowing how dangerous my syndrome was, I didn't know what else to do. I told myself that if he tried anything again, I would be prepared this time. But when I got to his office, I got a different, angry side of him. Gone was the lasciviousness: in its place, a temper. He told me I should get off all the antihistamines he'd had me on for years, the only buffer between me and the syndrome. When I asked him to clarify, shocked that he'd have me stop taking the medicine he'd been touting as the only thing keeping me alive, he shouted at me and demanded I thank him. He yelled, and the strange things he was saying were somehow scarier than when he had hit on me.

When I confided what had happened to a (female) doctor of mine, she put it plainly: "Don't go back."

To this day, I don't have a doctor to replace Valla. None of the doctors I've met in New York can legally prescribe my annual test. Every year that goes by and my levels go unmonitored, I think of all the women across the country who have been in this same bind: a doctor who harasses them, and no one else in town who can help.

Harassment like this, no matter how much we tell ourselves it isn't that bad, is enough to make a person feel unsafe. An incident also doesn't have to be sexual or angry for it to drive patients away from the only specialist they can find. Tina, the young woman with both PCOS and endometriosis, lives in a rural area, near only a few doctors. Few physicians in general specialize in the kind of endometriosis surgery she wanted to have, a procedure she'd been told would help her before she tried to get pregnant with her fiancé. So she was thrilled, she says, when she found that a doctor near her did have experience doing the operation. She and the doctor started to discuss scheduling. The doctor said he could probably do the surgery three weeks later. That sounded great to Tina.

"When are you getting married?" the doctor asked.

"Well, this is really our priority right now," Tina said—getting pregnant, she meant, not getting married. Her fiancé was thirty-two at the time, and she was almost thirty, and they knew that the surgery would give them a window in which to try to conceive.

"Well," the doctor said, "I just want to let you know that ethically, if you need fertility treatments—because of my religion, I will not help unmarried couples with any of that."

"Okay," Tina managed to say. She knew she'd probably need some kind of fertility treatment to get pregnant, given her two conditions. She left the room and cried in the parking lot. This was the only doctor in the area who could help.

Tina is an atheist, she tells me. She also believes strongly that doctors shouldn't discriminate according to whether their patients are married. But she was so desperate to have the surgery she needed that she tried to think of a solution as she drove home. She called the doctor's office. "This is a weird question," she told the receptionist, but what would the doctor need to see to work with her, to consider her "married enough" to help?

The receptionist asked the doctor and came back to the phone. "A name change will be enough," she said.

"I'm never changing my last name," Tina tells me when I interview her. "I have my last name tattooed on my neck in my dad's handwriting. I am never changing my name, even if I get married."

She asked a lawyer friend about the doctor's denying her care because of her unmarried status. If the hospital he's affiliated with is a public one, the lawyer said, the denial might be illegal. In the meantime, the suggestion was to find another surgeon.

"But I live in Bumblefuck, Wisconsin," Tina says. "I don't live in New York City or something, where I can just hop in a cab and find another doctor." In the end, she says, she went with the doctor who judged her for not being married. Luckily, Tina didn't need the fertility treatment that he maybe-illegally would have withheld from her.

In such a small town, she didn't have much choice.

———

In her memoir, *The Blue Cotton Gown*, midwife Patricia Harman recalls a patient named Penny.[12] The patient is thirty-seven and smells like cigarettes and perfume.

"I like coming to you," Penny says. "I'd rather have a female doctor than a man. You're nice."

Harman thanks her and decides not to correct her patient. As her name tag shows, she's a nurse-midwife, not a doctor. "I like helping patients take good care of themselves and making their exams as easy as I can."

Harman hands Penny a slip of paper with a prescription to help with her vaginitis. Penny takes the paper, but doesn't stand up.

"I don't like going to men," she says. "I had a bad experience with an exam once."

Harman is washing her hands, thinking about how to respond. "Was it a rough exam?"

"No, just the opposite," Penny says. "This was a long time ago, when I was seventeen." She pauses, seeing if the midwife is ready to listen. Harman sits back down and asks what happened.

Penny says she had just married her husband, Steve. They didn't want kids yet, so she was going in to get birth control. A medical resident saw her.

"He was young," she says. "Didn't seem much older than me, but all dressed like a doctor in a long white coat. He kept saying he had to examine me. He made me come back three times before he would give me the pills. 'I need to check your ovaries. They feel enlarged' is what he told me. He would tear the paper exam gown open real slow. I didn't want to keep going to him, but the birth control pills were free and I had to get them."

Harman hears the beginning of the story and knows something sounds off about the doctor.

"So I came back like he told me," Penny says. "The last time he locked the door, and the exam took a while. I don't know how long. The whole thing was so embarrassing. I just stared at the ceiling. He kept going in and out with his fingers. Touching me. I lay real still. Since I'd never been to a gynecologist before, or even talked to anyone about it, I didn't know what the exam was supposed to be like. I should have stopped him, but I was so shy. Now I would just kick him in the balls."

Harman pictures the resident touching seventeen-year-old Penny as he stands between her legs.

"I don't know how long it lasted," Penny continues. "Maybe ten minutes, but I had an orgasm." After the appointment, she says, "I was so upset I had to tell someone. I told my husband. He was only twenty, but he took me to the police. He said we had to do something, that the doctor should be arrested because it was rape. I hadn't thought of it like that. I'd felt it was my fault."

Penny and her husband went to report it. "It was awful," she says. "I had to tell the story over and over. More cops kept coming in and sitting with their little notebooks and writing things down. One cop told me it would be a hard case because it would be my word against the doc's. He asked me if I had gone to the emergency room to be examined for trauma so there would be proof, but there wasn't any trauma, so I hadn't gone."

Penny remembers the police making her husband wait downstairs. "I don't know why, *just procedure,* they said." She remembers hearing cops laughing out in the hall. "They took my statement and said they'd talk to the doctor, but nothing ever came of it. This was a long time ago. There were no women cops then. We were just kids to them, really."

Many women, like Penny, are ashamed or scared or minimize what happened to them. Many never report it to authorities. One young woman I meet tells me she was sexually assaulted during an exam by an ob-gyn that her mother worked with, one who even delivered some of her mother's children. "I was twenty-three and couldn't tell her," she tells me. "I still haven't; probably never will."

———

In 2016, the *Atlanta Journal-Constitution* published "License to Betray," part 1 of a series titled Doctors & Sex Abuse.[13] The writers, a team of journalists, list disturbing crime after disturbing crime: In Kentucky, Dr. Ashok Alur was examining an infection on a patient's abdomen—then told her that she had sexy underwear. Then, he rubbed her and placed his mouth on her genitals. The patient pushed him away and went to police.

"It was so beautiful," the doctor told her later, when she confronted him. "I couldn't resist."

And in Missouri, the reporters write, when a doctor named Milton Eichmann was supposed to be treating a woman for urinary problems after she had been badly injured in a sexual assault, he asked her "if she liked being tied up during sex, whether she was easily stimulated and whether she liked to be urinated on." Then he told his patient that he was aroused.

The report continues. A California psychiatrist named Mandeep Behniwal put his hand down a patient's blouse, grabbed her breast, placed his mouth on it, and then ejaculated on her hand.

One doctor, a Philip Leonard in Texas, had molested enough patients during exams that seventeen women reported him.

The list goes on. And in each case, the article calls the doctor by name to make a point: in all these situations, either the authorities conducted an investigation that seemed to confirm the accusations, or the doctors themselves acknowledged what they'd done. And yet, the paper found an alarming lack of repercussions for the doctors:

> All were allowed to keep their white coats and continue seeing patients, as were hundreds of others like them across the nation. . . .
>
> Society condemns sexual misconduct by most citizens and demands punishment. A teenage boyfriend and girlfriend in North Carolina were arrested for "sexting" nude pictures of themselves to each other. A Georgia woman was placed on a sex offender registry for having sex when she was 19 with a 15-year-old who lied about his age. A Pennsylvania teacher who had sex with an 18-year-old student was dubbed a predator and sent to prison.
>
> But when a physician is the perpetrator, the [paper] found, the nation often looks the other way.

How does this happen? The investigation found several reasons. Medical boards, dominated by fellow physicians, gave doctors second chances. When the cases made it to court, prosecutors dismissed or reduced charges so that doctors could continue to practice. And, in some cases, "Communities rallied around them."

The *Journal-Constitution* lists other institutions that have had sexual misconduct scandals on a scale that brought them to public attention: "The Roman Catholic Church, the military, the Boy Scouts, colleges and universities." All these institutions have promised to be more transparent about abuse. But the medical profession "has never taken on sexual misconduct as a significant priority. And layer upon layer of secrecy makes it nearly impossible for the public, or even the medical community itself, to know the extent of physician sexual abuse."

What prompted the newspaper to launch this national investigation was its research on a finding that surprised the journalists. In Georgia, they found, "two-thirds of the doctors disciplined in the state for sexual misconduct were permitted to practice again." When they decided to look outside their own state, the reporters found that every state in the country tolerated physician sexual abuse.

The series acknowledges that the vast majority of doctors do not sexually abuse their patients. Still, it found, in a parallel to the Catholic Church, "the phenomenon is akin to the priest scandal: It doesn't necessarily happen every day, but it happens far more often than anyone has acknowledged."

At the time of the report, in 2016, only eleven out of fifty states in the United States had laws requiring medical authorities to report to police when they suspect that a doctor has committed a sexual crime against an adult. In some states, the newspaper found, medical boards "cloaked sexual misconduct in vague language" or altogether removed public documents from online. Of the twenty-four hundred doctors the report examined for public discipline for sexual misconduct—again, keeping in mind that sexual abuse is often hidden or underreported—the investigators found that half of them still have active medical licenses. Half.

Philip Leonard, the Texas doctor who had seventeen women accuse him of molesting them during exams? The *Atlanta Journal-Constitution* investigators found that the medical board at first suspended his license. But when one patient who pressed charges went to trial and the jury acquitted the doctor, the medical board changed its mind. The doctor, as of 2016, was still practicing. What's more, the jury in the trial against Leonard never heard about the sixteen other women who had come forward. Instead, the group heard from the defense attorney, who attacked the patient's credibility when she testified. The medical board then decided to let Leonard keep practicing, as long as he saw only male patients for ten years. That restriction on him ended in 2014.

Some doctors who do lose their licenses in one state end up going to another state and practicing there. A former executive director of Ohio's state medical board, Aaron Haslam, told the newspaper that he grew weary of watching that happen: "It's frustrating now and it was frustrating then. We would try to be tough on an individual that we thought had no business practicing medicine and that individual would lose his license and go set up shop in the state right next to us or in Georgia or in Florida."

And the secrecy at medical boards that do discipline doctors but let them keep practicing means that doctors are not being treated as other citizens would be, as David Clohessy told the paper. Clohessy, the executive director of an organization called SNAP, which advocates for people sexually abused by those such as priests and doctors, put it this way: "Crimes are crimes, no matter who commits them. They need to be reported to and investigated by and prosecuted by the independent professionals in law enforcement. Period. Not a panel of your peers, not by some committee of supervisors, and not by other people who have earned the same titles you have earned."

The extent to which those in power choose to overlook a doctor's transgressions or crimes seemed to surprise even the reporters.[14] In Colorado, they write, a doctor named Louis William Bair had groped patients, made vulgar comments, and even had sex with patients—which the state considers exploitative and therefore prohibited. Despite these violations, the governor of Colorado chose Bair in 2002 to serve on the state's medical board, where, as the journalists write, "he could help judge disciplinary cases for other physicians."

The reports also found many more doctors accused of sexual misconduct than are listed in the country's only databank of such information.[15] The journalists learned that medical boards—partly because they deem each doctor an important resource to the community—sweep crime and misconduct under the rug.

———

Some women are especially at risk of physician abuse. Trans women who need medical care are up against a lot of extra shame and poor treatment by doctors. Victoria Rodriguez-Roldan from the National LGBTQ Task Force gives me an example of something that's not even direct—but certainly doesn't make the interaction feel safe. Sometimes, she says, if a new doctor doesn't already know you're trans, you might be tempted to not mention it. One day, she tells me, she went to see a pulmonologist. As she waited for him in his office, looking at the photos on his desk and the best-doctor awards all over the walls, she heard him in the hall. He was telling a nurse about a diagnosis that he'd ruled out as unlikely, since the patient was female and the issue was something related to prostates. "That's not possible unless there were some freaky Caitlyn Jenner thing going on," he said. The nurse laughed, as if it someone's gender identity was just a joke. Then he walked into the room to give Rodriguez-Roldan her test results.

"I nervously acted natural and pretended to not have heard anything," she remembers. She didn't say that she, like "freaky" Caitlyn Jenner, was a trans woman, too. She didn't need to feel derided.

The real joke, she says, is that the man being so callous and ignorant was located in what she calls the "liberal bubble" of DC—and a renowned doctor affiliated with a top university.

Members of the trans community in big cities are sometimes able to access care that's tailored to them. Practitioners at the Callen-Lorde Community Health Center in Manhattan, for instance, specialize in LGBTQ patients. They are trained and, presumably, are self-selected. A medical student who feels uncomfortable around people who defy gender norms probably wouldn't go on to work at a health center focused on trans patients.

And so, trans women who get medical care at places like Callen-Lorde are in a relatively welcoming environment. But ours is a vast country, and these clinics are the exception.

In 2010, the National Center for Transgender Equality and the National Gay and Lesbian (now LGBTQ) Task Force published the *National Transgender Discrimination Survey Report on Health and Health Care*, which at the time was called "the most extensive survey of transgender discrimination ever undertaken."[16] In total, more than 7,000 people completed surveys, and the final study sample included 6,450 valid respondents. Nineteen percent of those respondents—or about 1,225 people—reported being refused care by health-care providers because of their gender. Those who identified as American Indian or multiracial were refused the most. On top of being refused medical care, 28 percent of respondents were "subjected to harassment in medical settings," and 2 percent experienced violence at a doctor's office. An even larger survey by some of the same authors, in 2015, heard from 27,715 respondents. It found that American Indian, Middle Eastern, and multiracial survey respondents reported the highest levels of negative experiences with providers.[17]

Medical professionals lack adequate knowledge of transgender medical issues. In the 2010 survey, an entire 50 percent of the more than six thousand respondents said that they, as patients, had to teach their medical providers about transgender care. In the 2015 report, out of the more than twenty-seven thousand respondents, 24 percent reported "having to teach the provider about transgender people in order to receive appropriate care." This number still means that nearly a quarter of the people surveyed found that their provider didn't know how to treat them or weren't familiar with transgender people to begin with.[18]

In a 2016 report, the Human Rights Campaign—an organization that some think is too conservative in its fight for LGBTQ+ rights, but which is nevertheless a resource—recommended ways that hospitals can be better informed about transgender patients and avoid traumatizing them.[19] Its transgender-affirming hospital policies include making sure that hospitals listen to trans patients about which pronouns they use and ensuring that patients have access to helpful items like binders or padding so that patients can present as their gender while in the hospital. While some of these recommendations are specific to hospital settings and don't apply to everyday outpatient care, the report shows how simple some of the improvements in trans health care are, if practitioners are willing.

Even at the most trans-positive doctors' offices and clinics, however, there are still obstacles. Lea Rios, a thirty-year-old law student, has worked in trans and queer advocacy, including at the United Nations. She has reached out to let me know about the injectable-estrogen shortage, a problem that she says has affected many trans women across the country, including herself. (The shortage, I figure, has also affected people who take estrogen but whose gender identity is nonbinary.) When we meet at a crowded café and can't find any free seats, she suggests we head to her apartment a few blocks away instead. In her bright living room, we unbundle ourselves from our winter coats, and Rios heats up water for tea. As she goes to sit on a small, two-seater couch, I look around and realize that I'll have to sit in the only other chair, one whose curved shape I know will hurt my hip and back. But because Rios has let me—someone she has never met in person—into her home, I want to be polite. I decide I'll just suck it up and shift the way I'm sitting when it starts to hurt and see if that helps.

Rios takes a sip from her mug of tea and tells me about the short-age. Even at Callen-Lorde and other well-known LGBTQ+ provid-ers, she says, women like her couldn't access the injectable hormones they had been taking daily. The shortage got some press, but it was still affecting people. When she tried to find out from Callen-Lorde what had caused the shortage, it was apparent that the health center didn't even know.

Rios says she could instead take estrogen by pill, but she had tried it and it wasn't the same. It didn't make her feel like herself, and other trans women may have felt similarly. Paying a lot more for a private company that manufactured the hormone even during the nationwide shortage didn't solve the issue, either. Many cannot af-ford it. And estrogen shortage or not, Rios adds, the long-term health effects for trans folks taking the hormone have not been studied: an-other demographic that gets overlooked by research.

At some point in our conversation, my health history comes up. "You can see that my annoying hip problem still affects me," I say. "That's why I'm moving around a lot!" I say it in a too-bright voice, self-conscious that I've been unable to sit still as we've talked.

"Do you want to switch seats?" Rios asks.

"Actually, that would be amazing," I say. "Thank you so much! And I feel stupid, because I should have said something earlier. But I didn't feel I could ask you to switch seats, since we've only just met and you were so nice to invite me over."

Even though Rios has no health issues herself, she gets what I mean. Maybe, she suggests, there are similarities between our expe-riences. Having health concerns and needing accommodations but being too scared to take up space and ask for them seems parallel, she says, to being trans and needing accommodations but being too scared to ask, whether it be at the doctor's office or in daily life. Maybe, Rios tells me, we can start to expect others to treat us with kindness instead of being worried to ask for simple things. Rather than think it's amazing that someone would switch seats to help you have less pain, she says, "it should be weird that someone whose liv-ing room you're visiting *doesn't* offer to make you feel comfortable." Likewise, she says, we should consider it weird, rather than business as usual, when a doctor says or does something biased or rude.

———

Of course, many medical professionals of various genders are genuinely thoughtful with their patients. The majority of doctors do not actively harm those who visit them. But as the *Atlanta Journal-Constitution* writes, although most priests aren't rapists, either, there was enough of a problem and an insidious cover-up that the Catholic Church became known for the abuse scandal.

Yet even when doctors are ethical and nonviolent and kind, patients are up against a history of physicians and health researchers who neither understand nor even try to understand the needs of female patients. Many men and some women assume they know what women's experiences are like and base critical research and medical decisions on their own made-up ideas.

"If you go through the breast cancer literature from the fifties and sixties, before the feminist movement," health psychologist Tracey Revenson tells me, "it was so much about losing the breast. Femininity. Sexuality. Being a 'whole' woman." Now, she says, researchers are starting to listen to a different message from women: "Who cares about the body part—I want to lead a long and healthy life."

This isn't to say, Revenson points out, that all women going through breast cancer feel fine about mastectomies. That's certainly not the case. But, she says, "doctors thought it was all about the breast," seemingly without asking women what, in their lives, was important to them.

She remembers that volunteers from the Reach for Recovery program for breast cancer patients would meet women right after their surgery and say, "Here's a little wool ball right now—stick it under your nightgown." The push was to immediately give women false breasts while they were recovering. Starting in the 1980s, Revenson says, feminist researchers conducting evidence-based work found that women were saying, "I don't want to stick this wool ball in my nightgown—I'm in a hospital after my mastectomy, and I can be proud of my scar and the fact I am a survivor."

Audre Lorde, in *The Cancer Journals*, recalls this experience after her own mastectomy:

The woman from Reach For Recovery who came to see me in the hospital, while quite admirable and even impressive in her own right, certainly did not speak to my experience nor my concerns. As a 44 year old Black Lesbian Feminist, I knew there were very few role models around for me in this situation, but my primary concerns two days after mastectomy were hardly about what man I could capture in the future, whether or not my old boyfriend would still find me attractive enough, and even less about whether my two children would be embarrassed by me around their friends.

My concerns were about my chances for survival, the effects of a possibly shortened life upon my work and my priorities.[20]

And, Lorde continues, in a line Revenson is perhaps referencing during our interview:

To imply to a woman that yes, she can be the "same" as before surgery, with the skillful application of a little puff of lambswool and/ or silicone gel, is to place an emphasis upon prosthesis which encourages her not to deal with herself as physically and emotionally real, even though altered and traumatized. This emphasis upon the cosmetic after surgery reinforces this society's stereotype of women, that we are only what we look or appear, so this is the only aspect of our existence we need to address.[21]

Erin, the woman diagnosed with leukemia as a teenager on the way to the beach, mentions a similar story. Her doctor connected her with a wigmaker when Erin thought he should be focused on keeping her alive. She did end up wearing a wig, but she was pissed about the doctor's priorities.

We may have made some progress since the 1960s and 1970s, but some health researchers and physicians are still quite out of touch. Revenson talks about the women for whom the loss of their breast is indeed a really big deal or whose male partner makes it a big deal. There's much less research, she goes on to say, about gay women with breast cancer. Revenson once challenged a health researcher who had included lesbians in a study to explain why he had included them, since he hadn't asked them any different questions than he had asked hetero women. His response? "I got additional research funding for including them in the study."

Meanwhile, the US Office of Disease Prevention and Health Promotion says that lesbians are less likely to receive cancer-preventive services.[22] But the researcher had included them without learning anything useful, merely to get more funding.

In a piece about women "going flat" after mastectomies (something women of various sexualities choose to do), the *New York Times* interviews women who either opted not to have reconstructive breast surgery or had it and then after a series of infections or complications decided to have the implants removed. One woman, Geri Barish, the *Times* reports, said a doctor of hers had a strong negative reaction to her decision not to get implants. "How can you walk around like that? You look deformed," he told her.[23]

When it comes to autoimmune diseases, more than three-quarters of patients are women.[24] Some of these illnesses do get attention and funding for research, but others remain uninvestigated, relegated to a closet full of "mystery" illnesses that, as cultural critics and patients alike have pointed out, reek of the old misogynistic notion of hysteria.

"Research on 'women's ailments' is very limited," psychologists Martha Banks and Ellyn Kaschak write in *Women with Visible and Invisible Disabilities*, a handbook of sorts for therapists. Multiple sclerosis, they note, used to be called "creeping paralysis," and "was considered a mental condition caused by 'female hysteria.' It was not until 1996 that MS was recognized as an autoimmune reaction linked to viruses."[25]

Fibromyalgia is another disease still obscured by a cloud of "hysteria" accusations. About nine out of ten people with fibromyalgia are women.[26] In a 2004 paper in *Social Science & Medicine*, researchers observe that "in various studies during the last decade, women with chronic muscular pain such as fibromyalgia, and chronic fatigue syndrome have reported negative experiences during medical encounters: They repeatedly find themselves being questioned and judged either to be not ill, suffering from an imaginary illness or given a psychiatric label."[27] Women, however, were not only trying to be believed by doctors, or "struggling for their credibility," the researchers explain. "Their stories illustrated how they struggled for self-esteem or dignity as patients and as women."

Of note, too, is the title of the paper: "'I Am Not the Kind of Woman Who Complains of Everything': Illness Stories on Self and Shame in Women with Chronic Pain." Some women don't want to be "that" woman; they practice a version of self-policing in which they try to avoid becoming the stereotypical female. Regardless, doctors don't always listen. Some of the women whom the researchers previously studied showed that "hard work was needed to make the symptoms socially visible, real, and physical when consulting a doctor. Their efforts reflected a subtle bodily and gendered balance not to appear too strong or too weak, too healthy or too ill, or too smart or too disarranged." These women "organized pain and gender," as the researchers put it, hoping to prevent their womanhood and their body "from being used against them."

Chronic fatigue syndrome is the same condition Jennifer Brea discusses in her TED talk. Myalgic encephalomyelitis, chronic fatigue, systemic exertion intolerance disease: no matter what the name is, researchers have belittled it for years. A 2015 story in the *Washington Post* featured scientist Ronald W. Davis, who began to zealously study the disease only after his son, a young photographer named Whitney Dafoe, came down with it and could no longer function from day to day on his own.[28]

Davis tells the *Post*, "It's remarkable how insidious this thing is, in the sense that people who have it don't look sick, so nobody believes them." Most of the people diagnosed with the condition are women.

About his research, Davis says, "what we're trying to do initially is find a biomarker, something that shows a clear indication of something uniquely wrong." This, he says, "would help the patients a lot. It would mean that physicians could no longer deny that they're sick."

But when the *Post* ran the story, Davis, despite his position as a well-known scientist, hadn't yet secured funding from NIH to study the disease.

In 2016, forty-five researchers banded together to write "A Global Call for Action to Include Gender in Research Impact Assessment" in the journal *Health Research Policy and Systems*.[29] Here, the authors map out the many ways that women and women's health needs are overlooked in important research: "There is evidence that gender bias in biomedical and health research can occur at all stages of the research process." In particular, they found that "women tend to be significantly underrepresented" both as researchers and research participants in health studies. On the research end, although women reached 47 percent of admissions to US medical schools by 2013, they constituted only 38 percent of faculty physician-scientists—and an even lower percentage (28 percent) of these positions in the United Kingdom.

For participants in biomedical studies, the scene is bleaker. "For example," the authors write, "while women represent nearly half of people living with HIV, they are underrepresented in clinical studies of HIV antiretroviral drugs," showing up as only 19 percent of those studied. They are also underrepresented in what the authors call high-impact studies of non-sex-specific cancers.

And there's more. Female scientists tend to receive less funding for research than do their male counterparts, the authors write. That's important in a field where those with funding get to decide which types of diseases and demographics to study. Women are also underrepresented as authors of papers in medical journals. In some journals, the proportion of women who are first authors of studies—meaning the researchers whose names are at the top of the page before the rest (and whose names are often cited with the generic "et al." representing the other authors)—has "recently plateaued and even declined."

And, the authors write, when health researchers focus mainly on men and their experiences of illness, it can be harmful, and even deadly, to women. For example, medical researchers have mostly studied symptoms of heart attacks in men. Therefore, their studies haven't recognized that heart-attack symptoms can manifest differently in women. Doctors learned from those studies. So when they saw female patients with symptoms similar to those documented in male patients, the doctors gave the women the same types of diagnosis and treatment afforded to men. But when doctors saw women whose symptoms were different from men's, the physicians failed to recognize the symptoms or give them proper treatment. Many of those women died.

As the *Washington Post* noted in 2015, a report from the Government Accountability Office found that "NIH still isn't able to tell Congress—or anyone else—whether researchers are examining outcomes by sex to see whether men and women are affected differently by what's being tested."[30] Although scientists are usually required to analyze the results of their studies by sex, NIH has no process for effectively collecting that information. There's no standardized way to tell if a drug affects men differently from how it affects women. The *Post* gives the example of Ambien, which at the previous recommended dose "took longer to leave women's systems and could pose a danger the next morning." Once the FDA recognized the difference between men's and women's reactions to Ambien, the agency lowered the suggested dose to mitigate this health risk. When clinical trials fail to catch dangers early in a drug's development, agencies may only find out after it's too late.

Still, the rules have improved in the past few decades. As the *Post* explains, FDA guidelines from 1977 prohibited "women of childbearing age" from participating in drug trials at all. Not pregnant women, but any woman in the age range deemed childbearing. That ban wasn't lifted until 1993.[31]

Deena Walker, a neuroscientist at Mount Sinai's medical school in New York, studies sex differences in the brain. She tells me how she first began to realize how her own labs contributed to the problem of research that overlooks women. At first, Walker says, because she started out as a reproductive cancer biologist, she had done research on female rodents. But then, when she switched her field to neuroscience, the scientist who ran her new lab gave her instructions. "She told me to do my first experiment in males, because it would be easier," Walker says. "And I just had never considered what that meant. And then I had never really considered how many scientists just focus on males."

The idea that male rodents—or humans—are easier to study because they lack the hormonal cycle related to ovulation is, in current health and science research, "a really pervasive way of thinking," Walker says. Yes, she says, researchers are always looking for ways to have fewer variables. And hormones—which exist in both male and female rodents—have to be taken into account when an experimental subject is going through a reproductive cycle. In humans with ovaries, the cycle is roughly twenty-eight days, but in rodents, it's four to five.

What has traditionally happened in all kinds of experiments, Walker says, is that scientists use only males, and figure that females are just "smaller males"—that the results or effects they're studying would be the same in female subjects. That's been the assumption, anyway.

"I have a feeling you're going to tell me that that's not true," I tell Walker.

"And what we're finding now is that that's not true!" she says right after.

But, Walker points out, some of the social and cultural forces that go into this way of thinking are complex. On the one hand, early feminism was often linked to the idea that there's absolutely no difference between the sexes. On the other hand, as Walker says, "just because I say that males and females are different doesn't mean that I'm making a value judgment about one or the other. Females may take a different approach [in lab studies] because of their hormonal profile, but that doesn't mean the male way of doing it is better or worse. It just means that there are actual differences between males and females that are often regulated by hormones."

So as a feminist ("Can I call you a feminist?" I ask Walker. "Oh yeah," she says, "please do!"), Walker is trying to show that by completely erasing differences between the sexes in terms of bodies and brains and the chemicals that run through them, researchers end up counterintuitively working against feminism, because they overlook health issues that manifest differently in different bodies.

"Like what?" I ask her.

Walker gives me a concrete example. When hormones drive ovulation in a rodent, the rodent's behavior changes, presumably to make her more inclined to find a sex partner and mate. The shift in chemicals during ovulation makes her less anxious and more exploratory, Walker says. The hormones also make rewards—like sex— more salient. But not just sex: substances, too, are more rewarding during the rodent's ovulation. In the field of addiction, Walker says, it has been shown that "when a female [rodent] is ovulating, they'll have a stronger response to cocaine. Or they'll have a stronger response to alcohol."

That's in rodents. What about humans?

Walker tells me that until a few decades ago, doctors thought their female patients were lying about their substance abuse. Women (and here Walker is referring to cisgender women) would come in and say that they'd been using cocaine for only a few months but were already quite addicted. Doctors would think about what they'd learned from research papers. From their male patients and from studies in the lab, they knew it took longer than a few months for someone to become addicted. So they dismissed all the female patients as being dishonest about their substance history. Either the women weren't really addicted, the thinking went, or they were lying and had actually started using the drug much earlier.

At some point, Walker says, scientists finally introduced female rodents into their lab experiments. And, surprise: the results showed that women's claims of rapid addiction weren't lies at all. Women with ovaries had a stronger response to drugs and became addicted more rapidly than did people without ovaries. But until these studies with female subjects, Walker says, bias persisted—preconceived ideas that female patients weren't to be trusted, that they were conniving or tricky.

The score? Reason, logic, and science, 1. Misogyny and sexism, still 8 zillion. But it was progress.

Even during the past decade, Walker says, she has been quite unusual among scientists for studying female rodents. Only a few years ago did NIH mandate that scientists must now include females in experiments. But the mandate isn't a perfect solution, either. Scientists pushed back, Walker says, reminding NIH that if the institutes wanted researchers to double the numbers of subjects to account for two sexes, the researchers would need a lot more funding. NIH wasn't about to allocate that, so instead, its guidelines were a little fuzzy on how to meet the requirement. One problem, Walker says, is that as exciting as it is to now have to include females and not just ignore them as "difficult" subjects in an experiment, this new rule without a funding boost to go with it means that scientists will simply halve the number of males they include and add females. Consequently, the sample size of each group will probably be too small to show sex differences.

About the addiction researchers who started studying female rodents, I ask, what made them finally decide it was time to look at females?

To answer that question, Walker puts me in touch with Jill Becker, a researcher at the University of Michigan who helped pioneer the study of female rodents in addiction. Becker tells me that for more than thirty years, she's been studying estradiol, a hormone released by the ovaries, and how it affects certain brain neural systems that are important for motivation.

"In the early nineties," Becker says, "I was studying estradiol and motivation in the female, and seeing these effects of it enhancing motivation for a partner and acting directly on the reward system. And that's really my love, that's my main passion . . . trying to understand sexual motivation. I think it's important—and that's a whole 'nother story. But the short part of that story is really no one else is interested, because the funders are primarily male. And no one really cares if females don't want to have sex, because they can have it anyway." Cisgender women and other folks with vaginas don't have to be turned on to have sex, she says, and so doctors and funders don't put much effort into studying women's arousal or lack thereof.

Instead, Becker set out to find what might be of interest to male peer reviewers and those who held the funds for research. What could she look at that still excited her as a scientist, but that would also seem important enough to the men in power? She thought about the neurobiology of estradiol and other hormones that influence sexual motivation and mate-finding and realized that the same neural systems would probably make those with ovaries more susceptible to addiction, too.

"So," she tells me, "I put in a grant proposal to study this. And the first reviews I got back said, 'You're crazy. Everyone knows more men are addicts; women really don't get addicted. So this is not relevant.'"

This was in the 1990s? Yes, Becker confirms. The 1990s: her colleagues laughed at her attempt to study female rats and said that women don't "really" get addicted to drugs.

Soon, Becker learned that another scientist, a woman named Marilyn Carroll at the University of Minnesota, had published a study showing that female rats took more cocaine than did male rats. Since Carroll's findings gave credibility to Becker's earlier hypothesis, Becker cited the data, resubmitted the grant proposal, and got funding. Then she brought female rats into the lab. She found that female rodents anywhere in their cycle were more motivated to take drugs than males were. And once the rats had an increase in estradiol, a hormone naturally released right before ovulation, the sex difference in addiction became even more pronounced. Becker calls it the "subjective hedonic yumminess" factor: the time in a menstrual cycle when drugs feel best.

"How did you feel when you first struck upon what we now know is a correct hypothesis, and your peers thought it was a 'crazy' idea?" I ask. "How did that feel as a scientist?"

Becker laughs. "I've been bucking the system my whole life. So it was just another one of those, 'I know I'm right, and so I'm going to show them.'" But, she says, "every time I ask the question, 'Well, have you looked at females?' there's always this, 'Well, females are too *complicated*.' I've gotten that answer for almost forty years now."

That's from her fellow scientists. What about the doctors, the physicians who didn't believe their female patients?

When Becker gave a talk in the late 1990s in New York on sex differences in addiction, one physician stood up in the audience. "Every time I see a woman," he admitted, "I assume that she's in the emergency room because of aid-dependent children. And I assume that she's lying to me when she says she's only been taking cocaine for six weeks. Because it is not what we see with men."

Now that he'd heard about Becker's research, he said, he would reconsider his assumptions. Becker recalls that he said he would "start considering the fact that the women *aren't* lying to him, that in fact they really have only been using for a short period of time, even though their blood levels are so high."

What the doctor seems to have also betrayed in his thinking, I notice, is a bias against women who have kids and receive welfare or other aid. Maybe, by now, that doctor has unraveled some of his stereotypes.

I ask Becker about the bias she still sees in funding for health research.

"Every time that I submit a grant where I assume that people have finally *gotten* it," she says, "that both males and females are important to study, I get shut down. So for me, I feel like it's necessary to justify studying both males and females, even in this particular climate, where we're now *supposed* to study both males and females."

New NIH guidelines or no, she says, researchers constantly deny the importance of looking beyond the male sex.

———

When I visit Alondra Nelson, the Columbia University dean of Social Science, we get to talking about the problems with clinical trials and health studies. We discuss how they skew, to the extreme, toward white cisgender men, as in the studies that led to a disproportionate number of women dying of heart attacks.

"To what extent do we understand the experiences of marginalized communities to be universal and to be the big stories that illuminate something about the world?" Nelson asks. In general, she says, we don't. While it's getting a little better now, clinical trials have historically conveyed that white men can stand in for everyone else.

Meanwhile, Nelson says, nobody from another demographic is perceived as standing in for the larger population. Instead, "stories about women of color, poor folks of color, [are seen as] kind of curious and queer and specific, [so] as to not be generalizable."

In reality, from a scientific standpoint, a group of, say, all Latinx women and a group of all white men are similarly skewed. "They're both problematic, overly homophilic groups," she says. But in our culture, we view a group of Latinx women as too specific to be generalized to all humans, whereas we see a group of white men as the gold standard.

When it comes to heath studies, a lot behind the scenes influences outcomes. I speak with Katie Hail-Jares, a researcher who works with incarcerated communities, sex workers, and harm-reduction organizations and whose work often focuses on women. We talk about the kinds of studies that do and don't get funded and how the powers that be often decide to focus on one area that they think is useful to marginalized groups, even if it's not. She gives me an example. Many studies surrounding sex workers' health are about condom use, she says. But condom use is consistent: many sex workers use condoms frequently with their clients. So outreach from well-meaning researchers and organizations encouraging them to do so may be missing the mark, Hail-Jares says, since the health behavior is already happening. The data, though, show that sex workers' use of condoms drops off a bit when it comes to more regular clients—and then drops off further when it comes to their own romantic partners.

"So if we're coming up with interventions," Hail-Jares says, "it should really be around sex workers and their romantic partners." But that's seldom what harm reduction focuses on. "If you're not asking better questions," she explains, "you miss this other place for intervention."

In another example, Hail-Jares was looking at sex worker access to health care in Washington, DC. She wanted to know if they were, first of all, accessing health care, and if so, whether they were aware of resources that reduce HIV. She and her team asked participants if they were aware of PrEP, HIV medicine taken prophylactically to lower one's chances of getting infected.[32] There's been a huge rollout of PrEP in cities like DC, she says, and so, if health workers are doing a good job of outreach, those in high-risk communities should have heard of it by now. In DC, she says, high-risk communities include any low-income women of color, regardless of whether or not they engage in sex work.

So Hail-Jares asked the thirty-two sex workers in her survey, mostly trans and cis women and a few men, if they'd received any form of health care in the past twelve months. Of those who responded, 97 percent said yes, they had.

She asked the participants if they had received HIV or STI testing. Again, more than 90 percent said yes.

Then she asked if the participants had heard of PrEP. Only about 53 percent said yes. When she asked if the participants thought they were eligible for PrEP, just some 13 percent said yes. And even those who had heard of PrEP often didn't know what it was, with many participants thinking it was a local job skills program.[33]

They're seeing medical providers and getting connected to care, Hail-Jares tells me, and they're getting tested. And yet there are no conversations happening to connect them to an important drug being rolled out on a huge national scale.

The marketing for PrEP, Hail-Jares says, is focused on getting the medication to cis white gay men. And so, she imagines that health-care providers sitting across from a black woman in DC are not thinking about PrEP for this patient's demographic—even though, statistically, she falls into the most at-risk category.

"Here, I think it goes back to a gender bias," she tells me. "I think you don't want to talk to women about sex, you don't want to see them as at risk for HIV, even though in DC, the most at-risk category right now is cis women of color."

Even though groups in the area have made some effort to target cis gay men for the medicine, she says, at the time we're speaking, in 2016, there's been very little in the way of targeting cis women, especially cis women of color, very little targeting trans women of color, and almost nothing targeting sex workers. The drug that could help many at-risk women of color in a major US city is almost entirely being targeted at men.

Hail-Jares also says that queer women are vastly overlooked. While some would argue that women who have sex with women have low rates of HIV, the issue has to be looked at more closely. When Hail-Jares conducted focus groups with women engaged in sex work, she found that although many sex workers identified as sexual minorities—queer, bisexual, gay, and so on—in their work, they were having sex with men. While many people assume that female sex workers are heterosexual because of who they have sex with on the job (mostly men), one of Hail-Jares's studies found that only about 50 percent of participants identified as straight or heterosexual, meaning that the other 50 percent are likely to be queer.[34]

If health-care providers see a female patient who identifies as queer or lesbian, then they probably won't bother telling her about PrEP or other HIV prevention methods. But as Hail-Jares points out, this patient may choose female romantic partners or may even exclusively identify as lesbian in her personal life, but may sleep with men as part of sex work.

"I realize again, these are uncomfortable questions for a doctor or a tester to bring up," Hail-Jares says. "But I think it's also really problematic to have these assumptions and then not be offering, or not even be providing, information. How radical would it be if you just started offering PrEP to every person that you saw." If providers talked to every patient about PrEP, they wouldn't have to get over their fear of, say, asking someone who identifies as a lesbian if she's engaged in sex work with men. They would simply be asking every patient who came in, regardless of gender, sexual identity, or career, about PrEP. This open approach could help eliminate stigmatizing questions and awkwardly targeted conversations. And health-care providers would be helping the highest at-risk group for HIV, cis black women, get the information that is too often targeted only at cis gay men. There's a disconnect, Hail-Jares says, between what we know in the social services world and what we pay attention to in the research world.

What about her work with women who are incarcerated? I ask. Health care in US prisons is not good, but I'm curious just how bad it is. And women are the fastest-growing group in our country's incarcerated population, with roughly 1.2 million women currently in the system, including in prison and on parole.[35] That large number includes young women with health issues and disabilities.

If you think the health research on sex workers sounds bad, Hail-Jares says, the health research on women who are incarcerated is appalling. Statistics on the number of women who are pregnant or get abortions in prison weren't even available until 2015, she says: another example of how we as a society overlook women's health. And despite the often-abysmal access to health care in the prison system, for many of the women Hail-Jares has surveyed, it wasn't until they were in prison that they were first tested for and diagnosed with HIV.

But while, as a collective, we actively turn away from women and their basic medical needs and symptoms, we also scrutinize women and their bodies. Although disparities in health care and health research abound—and although institutions overlook women of color, young women, trans women, and women in general—there is also an expectation that we monitor women closely.

Tests like mammograms and Pap smears, writes medical sociologist and anthropologist Patricia A. Kaufert, "are a constant in all women's lives, an annual reminder that their bodies are under surveillance."[36] She writes about the near obligation the tests impose on women: "Their best protection—or so women are warned—is to agree to a routine examination of their bodies for actual, or potential, signs of disease and decay. Being screened is a duty; evasion is tagged as irresponsible behavior, a moral dereliction." Ironic, then, that health experts tell women they must submit to regular screenings and yet don't themselves study women's health issues nearly as much as they do men's.

The health research that focuses disproportionately on white cisgender men will hopefully keep shifting and becoming more inclusive of women and people of color. In the meantime, many young women will continue to fear discrimination, abuse, or just plain ignorance from doctors. Many women I met said they wished that all their doctors were female. Some said they made a point of choosing only women doctors. For me and for other young women, our wishes don't always line up with what's available. After one incidence of "not that bad" sexual harassment from a doctor, I'm afraid to be in a room alone with a male physician. But when I ended up diagnosed with thyroid cancer, I couldn't always choose. I needed a surgeon quickly, and I needed the physician with that eerie title of *doctor of nuclear medicine*. They were men. I just had to trust them.

Or, try to. When either circumstance or my insurance restricts me to male doctors, I find myself trying to cover my breasts by wearing a loose-fitting shirt or scarf. I know that, statistically, most doctors are not trying to harm their patients but are instead trying to help them thrive. Still, once a woman is made unsafe in a situation that had previously felt safe, it takes a lot to feel trusting again. When I find myself searching for boxier shirts and sweaters on the days I have doctors' appointments, I get mad at myself. Aren't I playing into the idea that we feminists fight against, that horrid blame-the-victim, she-was-asking-for-it framework? I probably am. I know that a doctor shouldn't harass or assault a patient, regardless of what she's wearing, period. But it isn't even fully conscious, my shift in behavior. More a self-protective measure that some part of my brain hopes will keep me safe.

# PART 5

# To Raise Small Humans—or Not

Danielle was just a year out of college when she pictured her organs leaving her.

Before she herself became a gynecological oncology surgeon—the one who admitted to me that she doesn't always believe her patients' pain—Danielle knew her mother had had breast cancer in her early thirties. Her grandmother, too, had had stage 4 breast cancer, and died. Danielle herself was about twenty-two when she found out she had the BRCA gene mutation, a mutation that increases the risk of breast cancer by up to 80 percent. To prevent cancer, as many other cisgender women with the gene mutation have done, she decided she'd have her breasts removed by the time she was thirty—and her ovaries removed by age thirty-five. That meant, aside from the terrifying prospect of losing parts of her body, she would have to speed up motherhood.

If it hadn't been for her looming medical treatment, she says, if she were able to hold on to her ovaries, "I am a hundred percent certain my husband and I would not have had kids in the next five years." Instead, she started the fertility process around age twenty-nine, knowing she had just a short window. "I feel *pressured* to have my children in the next five years," she says. Because she wants to carry the pregnancies herself, and because she wants to prevent her children from inheriting the cancer-causing BRCA mutation that she has, she and her husband have been doing in vitro fertilization, or IVF, where eggs from Danielle and sperm from her husband are combined in a lab. The lab then tests the embryos that form. On her first attempt, she learned that all the female embryos had the mutated gene.

"My mom thinks I'm crazy," Danielle says of the fertility testing. "She's like, 'It's not a lethal mutation.'" But Danielle knows her family medical history, knows what it's like to brace for disease, for a double mastectomy. "If I have the means to prevent my daughter from having this gene mutation," she says, "I feel bad to not at least try."

I follow up with Danielle about a year later. By now, she's tested more embryos in the lab and frozen some, including a few that don't have the BRCA mutation. If she decides to have kids in the next few years, she'd have one of the embryos implanted into her uterus and carry the pregnancy from there. Is she glad she went through all that testing, I ask, even though her mom thinks she's overreacting?

"Sometimes I regret it financially," she says, "'cause it was incredibly costly, especially for two young people who don't make a lot of money. We spent a *lot* of our savings on it." That said, she adds, she and her husband are both going into careers where they should be financially secure in a few more years. "If I didn't have that security," she says, "then it might have been a more difficult decision."

With her savings gone and some embryos frozen, Danielle is still not sure when she'll feel ready to have kids.

———

In her study of young adults who have had leukemia, Tracey Revenson, the health psychologist I met with at Hunter College, has found that women often don't have that kind of fertility choice. With leukemia, people often go to the doctor with symptoms, then find out they must have emergency treatment right away to survive.

"If you have acute leukemia, you're in the hospital that night, to save your life," Revenson says. Many young women she's interviewed said they asked the doctors about fertility options and heard a response along the lines of, "You have to be in the hospital right now. I'm sorry. I have to save your life."

In those cases, there simply isn't time to harvest a person's eggs. Still, Revenson says, many young women in her study talked about how little they were told by doctors about fertility options, even when they had less dire timelines and thus more days to take action. In many cases, she says, "nobody bothered to say anything about it." Whereas "men can freeze sperm immediately, before they start treatment," people with ovaries have to deal with a more complicated process. And so, she says, her research indicates that for young women who have had leukemia or lymphoma, there's an uncertainty about their future ability to conceive biologically. For many in their twenties, childbearing wasn't something they were currently thinking about—many were focused on finding a partner and starting a career. Now, after their doctors didn't talk about fertility in those early days after diagnosis, "they feel they were robbed of something."

Another issue that emerges in young women in particular is that when you're in your twenties, your parents may be more involved in your childbearing decisions than if you were, say, forty. Revenson says she spoke with a doctor who had a twenty-three-year-old woman as a patient about to go through treatment. The young woman's husband came with her to the doctor during her diagnosis—as did both her own parents and her parents-in-law. It was a scene. Both sets of parents were screaming at the doctor, "Save her eggs! We want grandchildren!" The husband was focused on what seemed most pressing to him. He said to the doctor, "Save her."

As for the patient herself, who had just gotten the diagnosis, she was simply in shock.


Many women with or without health conditions choose not to have kids. I happen to be one of those women. I feel relatively sure that I don't want to grow a child in my womb, mostly because of what my body has already been through. After missing out on that early-twenties feeling of invincibility my peers enjoyed, I can't imagine giving up the shred of autonomy I might hold now.

None of us has autonomy over our health, really. We just tend to think we do when we're young. And although my medical crises told me, forcefully, that all my young peers were wrong in their belief that they controlled their own bodies, I still want a scrap of their carefree feeling from a decade ago. Pregnancy, friends tell me, can mean back pain and skin problems and diabetes and bladder issues and pre-eclampsia. But even when a friend tells me that hers was a painless, beautiful, glowing experience, she admits that the pregnancy happened *to* her—that, as she swelled and shifted and grew, she wasn't really in control.

I want to keep whatever control I do have over my body. For the first time, after illnesses that kept growing inside me without warning, I feel I have a choice.

And although some women I've interviewed absolutely do want kids, they are quite aware of the extra loss of autonomy.

A writer named Natalie sends me her thoughts. She's a straight cisgender woman who has Lyme disease, arthritis, and a nerve disorder, among other things.

> I generally think of myself as having serious health issues," she tells me, after listing the many things her body is going through. "However, I do recognize that the fact that it affects my ability to conduct my everyday life does essentially qualify it as a disability. It's a tricky distinction, too, because there are 'disabilities' as real people see them and 'disabilities' as the government and insurance companies see them. So I think it's difficult for people that sort of straddle the line like I do to determine where they fit and to think of their issues as a disability since we can still mostly conduct our lives and often can't officially collect disability pay.

But, she writes, she does have to modify her behaviors and activities, and there are things she used to be able to do that she now can't. "So when I think in that regard," she writes, "I think *disability*."

No matter how she defines her experience of illness, she knows she has wanted kids for a long time. And she wants very much to conceive and carry children herself and raise them with a male partner. A few years ago, though, she was talking about these hopes with a pregnant friend of hers. "You have to get your health issues dealt with first," her friend said—and the reality of her friend's comment knocked her over:

> Because, as you know, when you have chronic medical conditions—and I have several different ones—they don't ever really get "dealt with." It would affect me drastically, with pregnancy causing more pain than I already deal with on a regular basis. I wouldn't want anyone to have to suffer daily pain the way I do, especially not my child and especially not because of me. I also wouldn't want my children to have to take care of me when it's my responsibility to take care of them, and I wouldn't want them to lose out on certain experiences and activities because I can't share them.
>
> But, with all those concerns, I still want a family. And I still want to have a child myself, carrying to term, if it's possible and safe, even if it will cause me more pain while pregnant.

As long as it wouldn't hurt the child, she says. Otherwise, she would adopt.

Natalie mentions that she has just had a round of intravenous immunoglobulin therapy, which helps treat some of her conditions. I ask if she'd have to go off any treatment or medication while pregnant. Is that why she's extra worried about the pregnancy causing pain, or is she just worried because pregnancy itself can be painful, regardless of going off medication?

"Wow, do I feel stupid," she replies. "LOL I didn't even THINK about that!"

"Oh no!" I tell her. I didn't mean to cause alarm. I thought she'd already looked into it since she has been thinking for a few years about the complications with children and her health.

"It's totally fine," she writes back. She's glad she's at least aware now. Now that she has looked into it, in what I imagine was a slightly panicked Google search, it seems that she could keep taking some of her medicines, but not others. Most of her meds, she says, including the ones she takes daily for nerve pain and for IBS, haven't been deemed safe, so she'd have to go off them. That change, she says, "would definitely cause an increase in my pain and discomfort, in addition to regular pregnancy pain." The good news, she finds, is that her IVIg infusions are actually considered helpful during pregnancy.

Considering all this new information, she says that she would probably still have kids, even if it means being in more pain—but she'd first test out what her body felt like without all those medications, "to see just how much pain I am in." And the level of pain "would be a major factor in my decision."

I feel bad that, like Natalie's pregnant friend a few years ago, I've hit her with another dose of reality. But that tug between which medicines a woman needs to take for her health and which medicines, if she's cisgender and plans on carrying a pregnancy, may hurt the fetus comes up often. As one eighteen-year-old woman in Australia tells researchers, "I know that they don't know really if lupus is [hereditary] but even if it isn't they could have kidney disease, brain disease[,] all these things from me. So I want to do IVF with a surrogate mother. Even if I don't pass anything on to them, my medications will harm a newborn; it is not something you want to burden your children with."[1] Another woman in the study, a twenty-six-year-old, says this: "If I fall pregnant, I'm on methotrexate that can actually kill my baby, that's what I'm scared of."

Tina, the woman with PCOS and endometriosis—the one who had a doctor discriminate against her marital status—was already pregnant when I met her. It had taken all kinds of effort to get pregnant and would take all kinds of effort to keep going.

PCOS and endometriosis can complicate fertility. PCOS can interrupt ovulation, as Tina has experienced. And endometriosis, which causes uterine-lining-like tissue to appear elsewhere within the body and can also cause organs to fuse, may affect fertility as well. Endometriosis can cause extreme pelvic pain and a host of other symptoms.

Tina had learned from doctors that "our best chance for conception was after my surgery, after I was all cleaned out." After an operation that "unstuck" her organs and fallopian tubes, she had six to twelve months to try to get pregnant before the health issues would resurface.

She also worries about having a miscarriage, which some believe might be more likely with PCOS. But even if she's able to carry the fetus to term, Tina is already concerned about wanting to breastfeed but having to go off the medicine that helps keep her conditions in check. "My biggest concern," she says, "is not being able to be on hormonal birth control, which means I won't be on anything to suppress the endometriosis from growing back." The adhesions that form, she says, are "like a blister. Anywhere those cells get outside your uterus, it's like a micro period. So the cramping that you feel on the inside of your uterus, I felt them on my fallopian tube and on my bowel."

About the baby's sex, Tina's thoughts echo Danielle's. "I go back and forth," Tina says, "but I feel bad saying it, but I hope that this baby's a boy. And I hope that—a lot of it is, I don't want to pass on all this crap to my daughter, cause it's highly genetic. But then I'm also like, it's just easier! Like, guys' lives are easier."

Unlike Danielle, who's testing embryos beforehand to avoid passing down the gene mutation associated with cancer, Tina got pregnant and is waiting to see what happens: what the baby's sex is, and what, if anything, the child might have inherited.

"I just really hope it's not a girl," she says, "so she doesn't have to go through what I'm going through."

Meanwhile, the medical community appears to be biased toward talking about fertility options with certain types of patients more than others. In a *New York Times* piece called "Is Egg Freezing Only for White Women?," Reniqua Allen writes about an older family friend, Ms. Rosalie, who reminds her that her "childbearing years were slowly ticking away."[2]

"A few months later," Allen writes, "after an unsurprising breakup, I looked at the fading surgery scar across my abdomen—the remnant of surgery I had eight years earlier to remove uterine fibroids and treat endometriosis—and realized it was time to heed Ms. Rosalie's advice. I started thinking about freezing my eggs."

But, Allen writes, even though egg freezing is becoming more mainstream and more commonly discussed, "few of the discussions are geared toward black women."

In the case of uterine fibroids, research suggests, black women may fare worse, with large fibroids and more hysterectomies.[3] And simply being a woman with an illness may actually correspond to a lower likelihood that a doctor brings up fertility options. Researchers surveyed 459 adolescents and young adults who were diagnosed with cancer in 2007 or 2008. As their 2015 study in the journal *Cancer* found, "male patients were more than twice as likely as female patients to report that fertility preservation options were discussed."[4]

And yet we women, in our everyday lives, are bombarded with the idea that we must want children or else something is surely wrong with us. Countless women have said to me, "You'll change your mind when you're older," or, "Oh, I used to be like you, but you'll see, it all changes when you hit thirty-five," or, "Don't you feel maternal, though?" and a host of other judgmental things. And then, when someone keeps asking me why I don't want kids, the person usually doesn't want to deal with the answer: that my insides have never felt like my own.

I have met other young women who feel the same way, who let out a laugh when they think about giving birth. "Not after what I've been through," a fellow health-issue-laden woman and I joked. It's not a joke, really, and yet there's some kind of wry humor we seem to twist out of it, something we use to counter the pressure to "glow" for nine months and give birth. I've always rejected the idea that having kids is a prerequisite for growing up. (Like those who choose to live single lives, people who choose not to have kids face stigma and the false idea that they're therefore not real adults.) Once my various health monsters stomped their way into my body, I felt even less inclined to become pregnant. Friends told me about their babies pushing on their ribs, expanding their hips, causing aches even in bodies without health concerns. I winced when I learned that a person's immune system gets suppressed during pregnancy so that it doesn't attack the fetus.[5] I can't imagine asking my out-of-whack immune system to do one more thing for me when it has already failed so many times.

Regardless of health, women have often confided in me, at parties, at bookstores, even at baby showers, that they're relieved to meet someone else who isn't bent on having kids. I know it's something people are often afraid to share. So when I'm e-mailing with Emily, the filmmaker with multiple sclerosis, and ask whether or how MS affects her desire to have kids, I feel oddly invasive. The question looks stark on my screen, less casual than it would sound in person or on the phone.

"Do you want kids?" I write. And then, to soften the question, I add, in parentheses: "I don't, which, since I'm a young woman, seems to freak people out, so I will certainly not judge your answer either way."

"I don't want kids," Emily replies, "but I knew that before I knew I had MS. I agree sometimes people freak out over that fact that I don't want kids so sometimes I'll just tell them it's because of MS. We still don't know exactly how people get MS, but if it is genetic, that's a great 'excuse.'"

Emily is not the only one who responds to people's pressure to have kids by armoring herself with her health issues to legitimize her decision. In a Reddit post titled "I Would Rather Have Lupus than Children," a woman writes, "I often use my lupus and clinical depression as the big reasons that I can't/don't want to have children."[6]

Below her post, a few women's comments focus on a combination of reasons. "Lady in my mid 30's here," one reads. "I have rheumatoid arthritis. . . . I was childfree before the RA diagnosis because I wanted a career. And now that the RA has taken that away from me, I'm EVEN more Childfree. GAH. I can't even imagine dealing with a kid while in a flare. Nope. Not a chance in hell."

Another woman writes, "i think pretty much any autoimmune disease should get people to take you seriously when you say [you're] CF [childfree]. but also they should just quit being so obsessed with babies and kids in the first place." In other words, it'd be great if we could stop telling women what they should do with their lives, regardless of whether or not they have health issues.

Vita, who, like Emily, has MS, tells me that having children can actually help people with the disease. Since pregnancy essentially puts your immune system on a lower drive, she says, so that you don't reject your fetus, her doctors have told her that women who end up pregnant tend to have fewer MS-related disabilities than do women who have the disease but are not pregnant. But, one doctor acknowledged, this doesn't mean that MS is a reason to go have a child. Right, Vita thought—"it's like eighteen years' worth of reasons not to have a child!" Her joke aside, she has always leaned toward having one. She does worry about her energy levels, but she hopes to have a supportive partner and dreams, as she puts it, of having cute little radical children.

———

Sophie, the scientist who grew up with HIV, has just finished telling me about how her adoptive mother, the woman she grew up with, was extra protective.

"My mom never let me go swimming, never let me drink water from the tap—I guess the bacteria. She always used my health status [to limit my activities]. I wanted to join the swim team, and Mom said no."

Sophie laughs at some of the claims her mother made. When Sophie first wanted to get a tattoo, her mom tried to stop her and made her ask one of her doctors. The doctor said it was fine. (She now has six.) Maybe, Sophie and I joke, some of her mom's concerns weren't completely about her health.

On one of the days we talk, Sophie, now almost twenty-seven, has just come from one of her many doctors' appointments. There, she asked if it would be okay to swim regularly. The doctor, unlike a certain mom years before, said yes to this as well.

"It's fine," the doctor told Sophie. "You can go about life. You can do everything other people are doing."

Everything. Sophie has already mentioned to me that she can have biological children. That she, a young woman who as a baby with HIV in 1989 wasn't supposed to live past two, can now give birth to her own kids.

But even though she can, does her health affect whether she wants to?

"So I—I think that I go back and forth," she says. "I do want kids. . . . I want that fairy tale of, you know, kids, at least two kids, and a happy husband and a happy life. That is what I want."

Later, she explains what might stop her: "I've always wanted children. The question, the real question, is, did I want to adopt children, or am I going to have children of my own? And I remember for the *longest* I kept saying I was going to adopt children." As a teenager, Sophie remembers, even when people told her she could give birth, she worried about the chance that she would pass on her HIV.

And adoption is meaningful to her, as she herself was welcomed and raised by an adoptive family. As a child who felt wanted, she tells me, she wants other children to feel wanted, too.

Still, she says, "the short answer is yes, I hope to be able to carry my own child. I would love—I have this idea about having my own blood child because I was adopted. And I got excited when my very own blood nephew was born. There's something about saying, 'That's my blood relative,'" she says, even though her adoptive family is more important to her overall. But Sophie knows how much work would have to go into her pregnancy and childbirth, how much more she'll have to do than others who get pregnant.

"I have to go on *more* medicine," she says. She seems honest with herself about her own habits. "I already suck at taking my medicine," she admits. The idea of a bigger heap of pills every day is a bit daunting.

"So for me," she continues, "accidentally getting pregnant is something that I pray will never [happen]. I try to do everything at all costs to not get pregnant before I want to. I want to get married before the baby, but I know that doesn't happen all the time." Sophie, who not only has HIV but has also studied it as a scientist, rattles off some of the additional things she and her child would have to go through. "I know the baby will be on medicine," she says. "I won't be able to breastfeed, I'll have to get a C-section. . . ."

But, she says, "I figure that if I find the man of my dreams, that it'll be easier."

Sophie is extraordinarily pragmatic and scientific; she is a person with a disease as well as a researcher of the disease. At the same time, she is also a woman who casually uses the phrase "Prince Charming." She wonders for a moment about how this perfect partner, this "prince," might make all the difference.

If she were to get pregnant without having a stable Prince Charming–type partner, she would have an abortion. That decision, she says, "probably is related to my being HIV positive." If she doesn't have a supportive partner, even though her family and religious community might frown on abortion, she doesn't think she would want to deal with the complications of her health and the pregnancy alone. She emphasizes again that for her, with HIV, the whole undertaking would require more energy and more medical intervention than usual.

"I don't want to get on more medicine," she says. "That's scary for me. The fact that you're gonna cut my stomach, the fact that many people have C-sections—"

"Why not vaginal birth?" I ask.

"Let's say the baby's healthy," she says. The fetus will be HIV negative. But, she explains, the mucus and blood as it leaves the canal could potentially transmit the virus.

"The question is," she says, "do you want to take that risk? All the money in the world," she says, and there's still a chance that your child will have HIV.[7]


Having a health issue or disability can affect the possibility of raising children in other ways, too. Victoria Rodriguez-Roldan, the National LGBTQ Task Force attorney I met for sushi, tells me that she and her wife want to have kids. Since she herself is trans and doesn't have a uterus, Rodriguez-Roldan would not be able to conceive. And since her wife, who identifies as nonbinary and who does have a uterus, has a connective-tissue syndrome, she might not be able to easily carry a pregnancy. The couple, then, might need to adopt. But adoption, she worries, would probably be hellish: when agencies find out about Rodriguez-Roldan's history of bipolar disorder, she says, "they're not going to want to give us a kid."


And what about this question: the extent to which a person will be "able" to be there for their child if they do choose to have kids? While it can be insulting, discriminatory, and even eugenics-tinged for people to challenge a woman on how she'll raise a child if she has a health issue or disability—whether it's mental health, like Rodriguez-Roldan, or what we consider physical health, like the women writing about their lupus and arthritis flares—some women do think about it on their own. Some worry that they will be too tired or will be dealing too much with their own bodies to help their prospective kids. It's a tricky subject. It's very personal for each woman making the decision about her body and the future, plus fraught, no doubt, with social pressure in both directions.

In *Voices from the Shadows*, Gwyneth Ferguson Matthews meets a woman named Moira who uses a wheelchair and has two children.[8] While Moira admits that she used to have nightmares of another woman taking her baby away and telling Moira she wasn't capable of taking care of her infant, she also says that when the baby is there, you just manage. You adapt.

"To leave my hands free to push my wheelchair," she tells Matthews, "I used to wrap her in a receiving blanket and carry her around in my teeth. Her body rested on my lap, and I just held the blanket in my teeth and wheeled. I even shopped with her that way, until she was old enough to sit in the cart. I carried her home like that, too, hanging my parcels on the back of my chair."

Matthews, who also uses a chair, writes that she thought this "a rather neat solution," but that Moira grimaced thinking about it.

"Other people didn't think so," Moira said. "They told me it was okay for a cat and her kittens, but not for a human mother and her baby." But Moira cared more about giving her baby the care she needed, not what it looked like to outsiders. She did what she knew she had to. She wasn't trying to serve as some kind of inspiration to nondisabled people, and she wasn't trying to get rude looks, either, from people who didn't like her method. She simply took care of her kids in a way that worked for her.

And that's what many of the women I've interviewed do: they figure out how to have kids or not have kids in a way that works for them. Some are pressured, by family members or cultural norms, to have children no matter what their bodies are going through healthwise or no matter what they envision. Others are pressured to *avoid* having children because of their health, despite their desire to have children. Most of the women I've met have stood up for whichever life they wanted—even as expectations of who should or shouldn't be a parent continue to swirl around them.

# PART 6

# Sick Like
# Miss America

When she was twenty-five, Meg's eyebrows disappeared.

She'd already found bald patches on her head in high school, when alopecia began attacking her hair follicles. During those years, while her friends strutted past boys, she covered her hair or positioned it just so and feared walking in the wind or running quickly. While at first it was her looks that she worried about—that everyone would see a woman with blank spots in her hair—Meg now worries, in hindsight, about her self-esteem. Looking different from every other girl in high school and, now, walking into a room as a bald young woman, she says, has affected her sense of self-worth.

When I meet Meg, she's out with a few friends at a bar. I can see that she's one of those people who always lights up the conversation, smiles mischievously when she gets to the punchline of a story, and makes her friends laugh. But when her body began to attack her hair, she tells me, it made her a different person. Before all that, she'd been curious about the world around her. She could enjoy activities, just like any other kid growing up. She could focus on things outside her body. But during those formative years in high school, and then when all her hair finally vanished at twenty-five, Meg stopped feeling like a whole person.

"I was so consumed by looking different, that I didn't think it was worth—or that I was worth—having interests or hobbies," she says. I can see her doubting herself. She is, however, one of the smartest, funniest, most fun-to-talk-to people I've met in a while. She sometimes seems to know this about herself—that she's sparkling and interesting—and at other times seems to not believe it at all.

Now almost thirty, Meg hasn't dated much. "I've never felt desired," she tells me. "Feeling desired by others is just something you need sometimes. And I've never had that."

As for her curiosity about the world, she says, it has been muted. She seems like a highly intelligent young woman who loves literature and film and trying new foods. But what is exciting for other people has become, from her perspective, less so. Being a permanently bald woman makes the world look gray. And a decade of feeling that she is "other" to everyone she meets has made her feel that it's not worth investing in herself.

"Every day, I get further and further from my potential," she says. She imagines aloud what careers she could have had, what higher education she might have pursued, had she not felt like a freak since high school.

When you meet Meg now, she has no hair on her head and nothing covering it. No eyelashes, no brows, nothing on top. Since she lost it all at twenty-five, she has sometimes drawn on eyebrows, but she has given up on wigs and hats and scarves. She is bare, and it is noticeable. She says she feels most acutely self-conscious at parties. Every once in a while, when she has had some drinks, she looks around, sees people coupling off or holding on to their partners, and she feels alone. In those moments, she says, she knows that because of her medical condition, her atypical appearance, she'll be alone forever.

She doesn't usually believe it when men hit on her—and sometimes, the men who do seem to be hitting on her are fetishizing her bald head. But in her early twenties, she learned that wigs backfire. Wearing a wig means that a guy might start kissing her and then realize she's bald underneath. It means mortification and shock. For her, the reveal is much, much worse than being seen as bald from the start.

Who can Meg look to as a role model? Most of the hairless women who come to mind on television or in movies are in chemo. Cancer—that's something Meg feels guilty about. Strangers tend to assume it's why she has no hair. Passersby sometimes whisper, "I had cancer, too. Don't worry, you'll get through it." Meg is not sick, though. At least not in the way they think. Alopecia is an autoimmune condition, but it's not, Meg says, anything at all like a life-threatening disease. It is humiliating and has ruined her self-esteem, but it's "not that bad" in terms of health.

One of the most recognizable bald women on television is the character Rosa from *Orange Is the New Black*. Rosa is older, dying of cancer, and mocked a bit by the other characters. When we first meet her, her skin is sallow. She wears a hospital gown while the others wear regular uniforms. She has no energy, and she's completely bald.

It isn't until the show's second season that we get to see more depth in Rosa: the wild, smart, "healthy-looking," gorgeous woman she was before prison, the devil-may-care attitude she had when she arrived. Still, most people see her as a washed-up older prisoner who has given up on engaging with those around her. Another character refers to her as "Mr. Clean." Bald Rosa is, for much of the first season, not only desexualized, but almost grotesque.

This image, of course, is not what twentysomething Meg is going for. It's what she's trying to avoid.

But one of the only other famous women in pop culture with alopecia—not from cancer treatment, but from the autoimmune disease—is perhaps too far in the other direction. She is Kayla Martell, a Miss America contestant from Delaware.

If pop culture is already sugary, the Miss America pageant is a Hostess cupcake factory. The event, which began in the 1920s, not only parades unmarried young women across a stage in a swimsuit and high heels and judges them, but also has a seedy history of racism. As Blain Roberts, author of a book on pageant history, writes for the *New York Times*, contestants from the South used to explicitly symbolize racist agendas, sometimes even promoting Jim Crow–era segregation.[1] For decades now, the contest has continued to promote "pure" young women's bodies. (Even if, as Roberts writes, the nude-body-hinting swimsuit competition has been repackaged as the "lifestyle and fitness" category.) It is all about shiny tiaras and looking telegenic on stage, or at least what's assumed to be attractive to straight white men.

Martell competed as Miss Delaware in 2011. One headline about her on the *Today* show's website reads, "Your New Miss America Might Be Beautiful—and Bald."[2]

Martell, who has participated in beauty pageants since she was thirteen, has "always competed while wearing a wig, though she prefers to go bare in her personal life." Indeed, she tells *Today*, the false hair is really just for the competitions. "When I'm home with my family," she says, "I'm always without my wig—that's who I am."

When viewers tune in to the pageant shows, however, they see her looking like everyone else: with hair.

For Meg—who, because of her baldness, often hates to be photographed, let alone nationally televised—alopecia is not "who she is." While Martell, a professional model, might feel that her alopecia is just part of her identity, Meg explicitly tells me that for her, it's the opposite. The lack of hair is utterly involuntary. And if she had it back, she says, she would wear it in "a wavy dark brown bun with curly tendrils"—just as she used to before going completely bald. She thinks of herself as very femme, and yet people she meets often assume that she shaves her head on purpose to look "badass." Her real self—her identity—can never be reflected in her appearance, no matter what she does. And she feels a particular kind of guilt when her personality is mistaken. She feels she has disappointed anyone who takes her to be punk, let's say, when she's not.

She gives me another example. A few days before our chat, she was at a discount department store, waiting in the checkout line. A young man at the store sidled up to her.

"Soooo," he said. "You have no hair! What's up with that?"

When she imitates his intonation for me, it sounds undoubtedly flirtatious. It's apparent from her voice that this was a guy who approached her in a warm, smiling, maybe even bashful way. A guy who found her attractive. But Meg has been so desexualized for the past decade that she refused to believe me when I say the man was into her. Her vocal chords could mimic his, and yet the rest of her could not recognize or fathom that that voice meant flirtation.

Either way, she says, situations like this are always hard. She feels guilty immediately at having to tell someone it's not an aesthetic choice, but a medical condition.

"Do you know what alopecia is?" she asked.

"Sort of," the guy replied. And then, as Meg tells it, he himself felt too guilty to keep talking to her. Too awkward for mistaking a medical condition for a style. He got mumbly, then walked away.

"When I'm in New York," Meg says, "people assume I shaved my head to be a badass. When I'm in the Midwest, people assume I'm sick. Neither is true. It's a triangle of guilt."

To other young women who are sick in ways that Meg is not, pop culture is similarly disappointing, if not more so. Meg says that despite all the guilt it produces, she does feel lucky that her disease isn't life-threatening.

What about young women who have to deal both with depersonalizing physical manifestations and with frightening mortality issues? For them, TV and movies—and, yes, even the Miss America pageant—imply an inextricable link between sickness and sexiness. Either you're a Rosa, with all your vitality and sex appeal lost to illness, or you're a beauty queen or Hollywood star, "defying" your health condition with your looks. There isn't much room in between.

Take another Miss America contestant: Sierra Sandison, crowned Miss Idaho 2014. Even for those of us who avoid the media froth around beauty pageants, Sandison's image was everywhere. In July 2014, a photo of her on stage in a bikini saturated the mainstream. From *People* magazine to NPR, it seemed no one could resist broadcasting their surprise and admiration.[3] What shocked them was rather small physically. In addition to a swimsuit, Sandison wore a small black box on one hip: an insulin pump for her diabetes. Writers couldn't contain themselves about a young woman risking everything in a beauty contest by wearing a medical device.

To be fair, Sandison is making a significant move by showing her medicalized body on television and asking us to still see her as desirable. She is, as reporters everywhere pointed out, helping young girls feel less embarrassed about their illness, their medical-device-saddled bodies. And that is something we definitely need. On her blog Sandison writes:

> At Miss Idaho 2014, as most of you know, I made the decision to wear my pump on stage while competing. That decision took me two long years to make. When I first started competing, I was using injections rather than a pump. I didn't want people to see a weird-tubey-machine-thing attached to me all the time, and could not wrap my head around having a medical device on my body for the rest of my life.
>
> Then, I heard about Nicole Johnson: Miss America 1999. She wore her pump while competing at Miss America. My whole perspective changed.[4]

Later, she writes, "An insulin pump doesn't make you less beautiful."

For someone like me who has in the past worried about how a weird-tubey-machine-thing would make others perceive me, even when it was temporary, I am somewhat moved by her honesty. But she is still a Miss America contestant. She is still talking about what is beautiful in a way that's relatively skin deep. Her postadolescent years center on winning approval and fame for her looks, on being publicly voted as hotter and, according to a very biased set of ideals, better than other women. In some ways, Sandison has probably helped others feel less alone. But she also inhabits an arena where white women, thin women, and femme-presenting women are elevated above everyone else. A woman of color with a medical device, or a women who looks more androgynous, just doesn't get the same praise.

Sandison feeds into the same narrative as her compatriot, the bald, wig-wearing Miss Delaware. The plot is simple, and phrased similarly in almost every story: This Young Woman Won't Let a Medical Condition Stop Her from Becoming a Beauty Queen.

By being part of a system plagued by racist and sexist overtones, even a well-meaning beauty queen arguably still helps perpetuate millions of viewers' body insecurities. And the story, with its idea that a young person who is ill needs to fight through it, to put on a happy face, and to succeed by cultural standards, also serves as an example of what some call *inspiration porn*. This is the term for the supposedly uplifting, two-dimensional stories about people with disabilities—stories that people without disabilities use to make themselves feel good, even as the tales reinforce biased expectations for bodies and how they should adapt.

Right around the time that Sandison's bikini photo bombarded the news, another image of a young woman with a serious illness went viral. News outlets and blogs on several continents shared the story of Bethany Townsend, a twenty-three-year-old from Britain. Among others, the BBC, *People* magazine, *Today*, and the *Huffington Post* told the feel-good tale of how Townsend—who has a severe form of Crohn's disease—posted a photo online depicting herself in a bikini. The difference between her photo and countless others, however, was that her colostomy bag was showing.[5]

Colostomy bags will never be sexy. For a while, I've used the phrase as a kind of shorthand, a way to describe the added pressure we put on women whose bodies stray from the socially constructed physical ideal. How the maddening expectations to look a certain way—the expectations that, no matter how much we discuss them, don't seem to be going anywhere—prove extra detrimental to those with a serious illness. A twenty- or thirty-year-old woman in perfect health already has too many expectations to measure up to. Now give her a disease or a visible disability associated with something taboo, like digestion and excretion, and her perception of being "less-than" is likely to get more overwhelming.

And yet Townsend's image was upending those social expectations. Her photo first went viral on the Crohn's and Colitis UK Facebook page: a slim woman in a black two-piece swimsuit lounging on a beach chair, all aviators and colostomy bag and tattoos. Countless stories described Townsend as brave. Most of them also emphasize her good looks—Townsend says she has done some modeling in the past—calling her a "stunning brunette," a "bombshell," and "sexy."[6] The message is roughly the same from each news outlet: she's still attractive according to mainstream thin-white-people ideals, even with a medical condition we're trained to feel a bit horrified by. As those mid-1990s Alanis Morissette lyrics put it, she's sick, but she's pretty.

Four women had already begun a similar campaign called Get Your Belly Out, but Townsend's own photo seems to have captivated the public far more. She has posted other pictures, too, some with her bag visible, others with her stomach covered by a top. About her modeling career, she says she's empowered to try it again now that people have so warmly received her image, bag and all. She was, until her husband took the now-famous photo, too scared to reveal her hospital-conjuring torso in public. Coaxed into wearing a two-piece, she says, she now feels more confident. Her husband and the estimated 12 million people who have viewed her image have helped. At the end of 2014, the *Telegraph* named Townsend one of the top hundred Britons of the year.[7]

Indeed, most press about her has been abundantly positive. But the British *Metro* writes that hundreds of people have "hit out at" the model, targeting her with comments that she's too thin, too unhealthy-looking.[8] As the *Metro* reports, Townsend is "too skinny" not because of an attempt to look lithe—something other aspiring models surely feel pressured to do—but because Crohn's disease itself often causes severe weight loss due to the patient's inability to digest food and absorb nutrients.

Of course, such an easily google-able fact may not stop people from lashing out at an extra-thin woman in a two-piece. And maybe that's not entirely their fault.

Townsend, in interviews, is thoughtful, caring, and a bit surprised by all the attention. She's moved that her husband's photo could encourage others with her disease to feel more confident about their bodies—their cut-open bodies, stomach-hole bodies, bodies with an embarrassing pouch hanging from it.

But we are accustomed to thinness, to the prizing of model looks. Sure, she's a young, striking woman with a serious medical problem, but she's also, to some viewers, only perpetuating unattainable beauty ideals. Only reminding them that they—whether sick or not—don't look svelte, or "classically" beautiful, or as fetching in a swimsuit. Even though Townsend's own thinness is due to her medical issues with breaking down nutrients, these viewers are used to plenty of other models who are dangerously thin because of cultural pressure.

The problem is bigger than Townsend—who does seem to want to lift up other young women who feel undesirable or ashamed of the trappings of illness. The problem—or one of them, anyhow—is that we talk about young women with medical problems in terms of how far they have or haven't fallen from good looks.

And our pop-culture depictions of women with health issues, not surprisingly, emphasize the virtues of staying foxy despite sickness. Illness is messy, but in Hollywood, depictions of even the tiniest hint of messiness, if we get such an image, often manage to still look tidy. That might be changing slightly, but in my memory from growing up, only one infamous image stands out. The first time I remember seeing a young, vibrant woman who was seriously ill on television was 1998, when the then-new series *The Real World* was a hit on MTV. On the reality show, Irene, one of the residents, is acting strange. She appears erratic and out of control and decides to leave the show. Some of her housemates attribute her behavior to her Lyme disease. Years later, Irene, the real Irene, tells *New York* magazine's *Vulture* that she left because she hated being on a reality show where everything was fake and manipulated behind the scenes. "Instead," she says, "the narrative was that Lyme disease was making me delusional, which was unfair and cruel: Unfair to people with Lyme disease, and cruel to me."[9]

That narrative was so memorable, in fact, that when I was diagnosed with Lyme, a montage of scenes with Irene floated back into my mind. I thought, "Wait, isn't this the illness that makes you act all out of control?" Then I realized: my impression of Lyme disease as a "crazy woman's" illness stemmed almost entirely from watching MTV fifteen years earlier.

Judy Z. Segal, a scholar who has analyzed the language around body image and medicine, writes in one paper about "movies like *Why I Wore Lipstick to My Mastectomy*, videos like *Crazy Sexy Cancer*, and television shows like *Desperate Housewives, Sex and the City,* and *The Big C.*" In these popular narratives, she writes, "women with cancer are now encouraged/expected to be not only upbeat and positive but also sexy, and ready for sex."[10] She calls this trend "the sexualization of the medical subject." And she has found that the act of sex itself has become "the comic ending of the illness narrative."

But as we can see from Townsend's modeling and the Miss America contestants, the theme isn't limited to fiction. One contributor to *People* magazine wrote jointly about Sandison and Townsend as women who are changing our perceptions of beauty. He ends the piece saying, "I hope that more people with inner beauty speak out about their beautiful—and inspiring—imperfections."[11]

But in case it isn't obvious enough: we make these sick-but-still-beautiful women famous specifically because of their outer beauty, not really their inner. You don't find the internet blowing up with "inspiring" tales of a woman who uses an insulin pump and who wears a larger clothing size, or whose face doesn't meet certain skewed ideals. Not to mention that all these women appear to be white.

While dealing with health can be hard no matter what your identity is, dealing with the public scrutiny around it is easier for those who are white, straight, and cis. As comedian Wanda Sykes puts it in a reveal of her cancer diagnosis on the *Ellen* show, "I was like I don't know, should I talk about it or what? Because I mean, how many things could I have, you know: *Black*, then you're a *lesbian*"—here, the audience laughs as she piles up the minority groups and looks exhausted. "And I'm like, I can't be the poster child for *everything*."[12]

And when it comes to cancer, some have pointed out how harmful the popular narrative can be. A *Slate* piece from 2013 makes it clear in one headline: "Stop Demanding Positivity from Cancer Patients."[13] In the journal *Literature and Medicine*, Judy Z. Segal writes about the responses readers sent her after she published an op-ed in the *Vancouver Sun* titled "Cancer Isn't the Best Thing That Ever Happened to Me."[14]

Segal and others who have had cancer find that the popular idea that they must be "positive and pink-minded" becomes a burden. They feel that cancer is not an enriching, ennobling experience, contrary to many popular narratives, and that among other things, there are such strong expectations around how people with cancer should behave, there is "little space to tell, or hear, the truth about the experience of illness."

In a poem published in *Birdfeast* magazine, writer Daniela Olsze-wska gets at these expectations:[15]

*EveryoneHasToBe*
*NiceToYouIfYou'reSick . . . Un-*
*LessYou'veCaughtTheBrand*
*OfSickThatTakesTooLongToGet*
*WellSoon.*

Katherine Russell Rich, in her essay "A Mass for Katherine," which describes her editor's aversion to deathyness, also discusses the popular narratives around illness. "I was still fuzzy," she writes, "on the four types of cancer: magazine, movie, television and actual fact."[16] She writes that in magazine stories, "chemo makes women plucky." Television cancer, however, is "two hours of platitudes and exacting makeup" and doctors "with good hair. Everyone hates it because it's a lie." And in some ways, she implies, being bombarded with these tidily packaged cancer stories doesn't prepare us for the difficulties of the real thing, including having our lumps ignored by doctors and being told by everyone we encounter that we're too young to have the disease.

As much as Rich's wry descriptions feel spot-on to me, perhaps some of the tropes she describes do help some women. Maybe the popular narratives aren't always harmful. A magazine piece that shows someone being "courageous" during chemo might feel like sanitized inspiration porn to many of us—but it might help others feel more determined while facing their own illness, and at that, maybe we shouldn't roll our eyes. That said, the cancer patient on television with perfect makeup and Hallmark-card quotes flying around doesn't seem to help much. Neither does a scene where a celebrity looks ef-fortlessly beautiful while she goes through something that in reality makes you exhausted and full of nausea. To think that screenplays written or approved by cis white men can provide respite from the de-mands on female bodies is to forget what world we live in.

A celebrity who might actually be helping is comedian Tig Notaro. In the fall of 2014, Notaro bared her breasts on stage. That is, she bared the lack of them. The *New York Times* and others published stories right away: a woman showing her mastectomy to a huge audience, daring them to watch while she continued doing stand-up not just topless, but visibly scarred.[17]

The way that she visually conveyed a kind of "Hey, guys, my breasts were lopped off, and I'm still a person" thrilled me. It thrilled a lot of people, and it moved a lot of them, and in the mathematics of gender and illness representation in pop culture, it's a positive sum.

I speak with Beza Merid, a scholar who has studied stand-up comedy and the popular culture of cancer, and whose dissertation focused in part on Notaro. He explores how people like her challenge the popular rhetoric around cancer and so-called survivor status. He echoes what health researchers, Audre Lorde, and others have said: "After radical mastectomies, women often times are pressured to or feel pressured to have reconstructive surgery, [and to think] that mastectomied bodies are to be 'repaired.'" Notaro resists that pressure. She is also, Merid tells me, one of the comedians who is sharing her life much more intimately than comedians a few decades ago ever did.

One of Notaro's comedy tours is called "Boyish Girl Interrupted." Although she certainly surprised her audience with her topless, scar-baring moment, she is, as the tour title suggests, more butch than femme. That shouldn't matter, but in our femme-obsessed culture—where even a thin woman who wears dresses gets scorned and side-eyed by peers when she doesn't don makeup and heels for a job interview (which I've experienced firsthand)—it does. Notaro's act blasted through some of our unhealthy ideas of gender and illness, but the reaction probably would have been different if she were a straight femme woman. By already being "boyish," she might not have elicited the same level of shock—and even audience disgust—that a very "feminine"-looking breast-scarred woman on a stage might have provoked. It helps that she's already queer.

Lena Dunham is another celebrity who has opened up in a raw way about her health. Dunham became famous for her film *Tiny Furniture*, for the television show *Girls*, and, generally, for showing women as having sex drives and art projects of their own rather than being docile playthings for men. More recently, she has written about her experience with endometriosis and recorded doctors' visits for her podcast. She talks about the extreme pain that endometriosis gives her and the false assumptions doctors make. "The stigma around the reproductive system is part of why I'm so obsessively polite to nurses, doctors, and wheelchair pushers," she says in an episode. "Maybe, with the correctly sunny disposition, I can show them beyond a shadow of a doubt that I'm not here on a mission for drugs and sympathy. I just want to get back to work."[18] She lets the audience listen in on her trip to the emergency room, and she talks about the strangeness of vaginal ultrasounds. She's honest about how frustrating a disease endometriosis is, how it's messy and often needs surgery and generally sucks.

And Selena Gomez, who made her lupus diagnosis public a few years ago after taking a break from her career as a pop singer and actress, has also been up-front about some of her less glossy symptoms. "I've discovered that anxiety, panic attacks and depression can be side effects of lupus, which can present their own challenges," she said.[19]

But although a few famous women have shared the unvarnished experiences of their bodies, our television and film and cheery-news-segment images rarely line up with the realities of being a young woman with health issues. As writer Eliza Berman puts it in *Slate*, "sick lit" and "sick flicks" usually follow the same predictable arc and sugarcoat what illness is really like. In these hetero love tales, Berman writes, "a man or boy who's got his values all out of whack— he's a bad boy, or a womanizer, or a workaholic, or all three—falls for a woman or girl who's different from his usual type. Quirky, free-spirited, and possessing a wisdom beyond her years, she initially rebuffs his advances but eventually relents. The peak of their love affair coincides with the beginning of her demise, and in her graceful dying she teaches him how to truly live."[20]

The 1970 film *Love Story*, Berman points out, established the potential for movies in this mold to succeed, and films like *A Walk to Remember* and *Sweet November* followed in its saccharine path.

"Of the unnamed affliction that ails Ali MacGraw's character in 'Love Story,'" Berman writes, "Roger Ebert wrote that its 'only symptom is that the patient grows more beautiful until finally dying.'"[21]

———

Glamorizing "brave" young women who defy their diseases, or "graceful" women who act as catalysts for the men around them, probably doesn't help us much. Too often the characters we see reduce a woman's experience to a convenient notion: that her body is her own problem to overcome or that she must accept her fate with a smile—and that she is morally better if she does so while looking mainstream beautiful.

In writing this book, I have realized that while this kind of "bravery"-filled inspiration porn has always made me bristle, as it does many people with a disability, I have been avoiding thinking of myself as just that: someone with a disability. My health issues aren't tidy—not just cancer, not just autoimmune, but a tangle of things, some bendy twigs and a strip of plastic and a strand of hair and some wire that the bird of me gathered in its beak when I wasn't looking, then arranged in a frustrating nest.

"Are you a person with a disability?" someone asks, and I think, No, I'm just all these weird, hard health things woven together.

A number of people I've interviewed have gently pointed out that a disability doesn't have to look like the one clean narrative we see in movies or on feel-good shows, the kind where a person using a wheelchair smiles and reassures everyone that she's fighting the good fight. We have these images in our heads of what disability looks like and what counts. But many of the women I've met have made me realize that disability is largely about the world's failure to make space for you—and that it can be connected to a combination of things your body does, or an invisible syndrome or disease, or a hard-to-summarize history of surgeries. It need not be as two-dimensional as it looks on TV.

Okay, I think. Maybe I'll try on the idea that I don't just have health issues, but that I have a mesh of disabilities. In an e-mail I write to someone, I have to quickly describe the perspective I'm coming from in my research: "a queer woman with several physical disabilities," I write. It looks funny to me, but also accurate. It reminds me of the first time I used the words *gay* and *queer* in reference to myself. It was true, I knew it was, but was I "allowed" to define myself this way? All these terms at first made an uncomfortable heat crawl up the back of my neck. I felt transgressive, embarrassed, and proud all at once. I couldn't tell how much of it was internalized stigma. Being part of both groups, people who are queer and people who are disabled, wasn't necessarily up to me. It just *was*. But even if it was beyond my control that I was gay, that my hip became painful when I sat for too long, and that I had a scar where my thyroid used to be, claiming those identities seemed like a scary step.

Now that the women I've interviewed and the essays I've read have closed the distance between my experience and the word *disability*, though, doesn't mean that the word can fully capture what many young women and I have been through with our bodies. Having come within a few seconds of dying when I was just twenty-two, I still don't know how to categorize that experience. There, *disability* doesn't cut it. My body, which I'd like to keep frolicking around in for a while, closed its own throat and hurtled its own blood pressure down. What does that kind of thing do to a young person?

Pop culture often tells us that people who've gone through near-death experiences wake up and feel suddenly more alive and seize-the-day-y than they ever have before. We're supposed to reevaluate everything and change forever, according to movies and television. Drop off the grid completely and hitchhike around the country, climb Mount Everest, or just generally give no fucks.

A little while after my anaphylaxis episodes in New York and then India, my boss asked how I was doing. She'd just watched an episode of a TV show, she said, in which one character, a young woman, had had a near-death experience. But instead of going full carpe diem, the woman on the show had said, she'd found that the whole live-every-day-as-if-it's-your-last impulse is there at first, but wears off over time. Especially once she realized that still being alive means still doing small, everyday things: picking up a pineapple at the grocery store. Putting a rent check in the mail.

"Was the TV character right?" my boss asked. Was the seize-the-day stuff not as mind-blowing as people say it is?

"Sort of," I told her. I was now more acutely aware that at any minute, your body could stop functioning and that maybe it would be good to make sure every moment was meaningful. So some of that carpe diem stuff was in me, for sure. But I was also aware that, as the character said, this feeling can fade a lot or get eclipsed when you remember the responsibilities and the realities of your everyday life. I certainly felt different, and something had shifted that would probably never shift back. I now thought of myself as less invincible than other people my age. But the regular stuff of daily life hadn't magically disappeared. I didn't suddenly need to scale a mountain. I did, though, think more about how I spent my time and energy: more hangouts with friends on a whim, (slightly) fewer panics about work deadlines. Whereas eating a burrito hadn't been all that unusual for me before, I was now thrilled to eat one—and all the other foods I hadn't been allowed during my allergy testing, when I'd gone to that mediocre restaurant on a date and had ordered a bland omelet for dinner. I wasn't going to ditch all of modern life and live in the woods or suddenly ditch this job right now and find myself, but I was going to finish out the next year of the position and then take time off to focus on my writing career.

I was seizing the day, I suppose. Just in less grandiose ways than in most movies. That one depiction my boss had seen on television did, in many ways, ring true.

Still, bodies and health are messier and more varied than what we see on TV. So is being a woman. Maybe the ways women with health issues move through the world, the everyday world, will start to become more visible.

As Simon put it, we are all a riot wrapped in skin. And like the character whom Roger Ebert critiques, we are all on our way to finally dying. Not just those with health issues or disabilities. Not just women, either. Perhaps we'll begin to choose for ourselves what it means to do so beautifully.

# ACKNOWLEDGMENTS

Thank you, first and foremost, to the women who shared a piece of themselves for this book. I could not have written this without your openness, your insights, and your willingness to talk with a stranger about hard and complicated and sometimes funny-sad things. Thanks for the "Oh man, the same exact thing happened to me!" moments, as well as the moments where we learned about our many differences. For those whose stories appear in these pages, I hope I've captured at least some of the spirit of your experience.

And thank you to the rest of the team that made this book possible. To my editor, Helene Atwan, director of Beacon Press, who helped guide this idea until, incredulously, it became a book, and to everyone at Beacon who answered my questions, reviewed and copyedited and proofread and laid out the pages, designed the cover, and made sure lots of readers learned about this project.

To my agent, Jess Regel, one of those badasses you can count on to be calm, poised, and ready for the next thing, even when faced with a panicked writer. Thanks for sticking with this no matter what—and for being there when shit got real.

To all the strangers I met who said, "Hmm . . . I think I know someone who'd be good for your research," and who ended up putting me in touch with incredible sources. Thanks, too, to HARO, for connecting me with three women and their stories.

To Andi Bartz, for those all-important words, which went something like this: "That sounds bigger than an essay. That sounds like a book." If it hadn't been for our conversation, I might not have written this at all. (Even if it did take me a few years to believe you.) Thanks, friend. And thanks for your thoughtful edits and essay swaps over the years.

To David DeVries, recently retired dean at Cornell, for taking me seriously when I was seventeen. Thanks for making sure I was not just an English major, but proud of it.

To Lydia Fakundiny, who I wish were still alive so that I could thank her for being one of the best teachers I've ever had, and whose class I still think about thirteen years on. Thank you for pushing me to examine language in new ways and for being open to changing your own mind when little undergraduate me suggested a new idea. And sorry for all the times I use "so" the way you warned us not to. I hear your voice often when I write.

To the New York Public Library, for furnishing me with the volumes I needed and a semi-secret room to work in. Thank you for helping me begin my research as a Wertheim writer-in-residence and for filling me with the same awe I felt as a kid each time I walked into my local branch.

To my fellow members of Columbia's NeuWrite group, for workshopping chapters, cheering me on, and asking great questions that we didn't always have the science to answer. A particular shout-out to Caitlin Shure for helping me access the studies I needed and for distracting me with fun science history.

To the Tent Creative Writing community, especially Josh Lambert, for a snazzy fellowship experience, late-night conversations, and tons of support.

To Jenny Xie, fellow poet-who-constantly-revises-lines. Thanks for helping a new friend with one of the most important ones!

To Erika Jo Brown, for keeping it real in the poetry world. Thanks for your no-b.s. approach to readings.

To Tamara Garvey, for pointing me to Samantha Irby's blog, and to Freddie Bepler, for pointing me to Samantha Kittle's blog. Thanks, friends, for making this book more robust.

To Will Swanson, who might not know it but whose evolving thoughts on bodies and health helped me think about my own. Thanks, too, for cracking me up.

To Alana Staiti, who gave me a helpful zap of academese. Thanks for sending me smart things, and for being the kind of friend I can call in a word emergency.

To Patrick Hegde, for puns and for hearty talks and for always offering to lend a hand. Thanks for being snazzy and for always being there, which looks cheesy written out but is true. Let's hope that by the time you read this, we've finally gotten that dosa.

To Rachel Wasser, for keeping me on task. There's nothing like having a Rae Rae sitting across from you to make sure you get things done between seltzer breaks.

To Laura Silver, for zeal and wisdom and hilarity, and for understanding my writer brain. Also, for knowing that it takes just two good friends to make a conference happen anywhere. Thanks for helping me feel less overwhelmed in book city. Train-ride symposium soon?

To JAMSAM: you know who you are and you (hopefully) know how much I heart you guys. (And here's to JAMSAM's debut in the Library of Congress! Maybe some future archivist will decide that it's a very important term.) Thank you for all these years of friend love.

To Osmun: all of ya. Upstairs and down-. Who else would I make fun of everything with, or dance with on the spine of a thirty-year-old couch? Thank you for being a big fun sprawling friend family, and for being just as good at talking through the hard stuff as our long-ago selves were at throwing ragers.

To Maritza Jean-Louis, for getting it. Always. Thank you for being you. I'm beyond glad that we have each other.

To Alex Berke, for cheering me on and for having way more excitement about the long publishing process than I could have mustered myself. Thank you for bringing your ATB sparkle to everything and for making me feel like I got this.

To Benno Kling, for dropping everything to brainstorm subtitles, take photographs, even read and edit a whole draft. For telling me that I make good sentences when I said, "Aaaahhh I can't write this book / how am I going to write this book / aaaahhhh!"—and for giving feedback that you thought was too much when in fact it helped make this much better. Thank you for being an excellent unofficial writing shrink, and for pulling me up.

To Michael Jacobs, for taking me to the hospital despite my saying I was fine. Thank you for realizing that every moment mattered, and for making sure I didn't actually turn ghost. To Kate Black, for staying vigilant over me while we tried to stay vigilant about the country. Thank you for that whole adventure in 2008—the best way to become friends—and for keeping me safe that day. And to Smita Ghosh, for too much to list here: you maybe don't realize just how much it says that you not only stopped a train for me but then stayed with me every night squished on that hospital-room couch to make sure that I survived. When we met back in bio class as newly minted teenagers confused about microscopes, we couldn't have predicted all that. But none of it is surprising. You've been an incredible friend to this fish since the start—one who understands my little heart, whether in an emergency or just while talking till late about something hard. So: thank you each for helping to save my life. You all mean a lot to me, either way, but the whole not-letting-me-die thing doesn't hurt. And, clearly, I don't know how to write about it here without making jokes—it's just a little overwhelming to owe my aliveness to you. Thank you, each of you, for nothing short of everything.

To Bailey Georges, who has one of the loveliest brains I've ever had the honor to storm with. Thank you for helping me think through dilemmas big and small, for being a thoughtful creature as you edited a draft of this book and made it better, for drawing me that purring insect and sensing when things were hard. Thank you for being just as meta as I am, for letting us constantly laugh at ourselves, and for sharing your brainheart with me.

To Jane Isay, whose guidance and wit and friendship have buoyed me for the past few years, and from whom even the phrase "You need to redo this part" ends up feeling like a warm hug. I cannot thank you enough for encouraging me to make this book happen, and am so glad we happened to meet and talk about death and crappiness that day. Thank you for being a wonderful human.

To all of the Deslooveres, for helping me become the Mich that I am today. Thanks (ganks) for many a year.

To Elaine Joannides, for being part of the family. Thank you for all these years of love, and for showing up at the hospital on two very different days.

To Lillian Lent, for being a wonderful aunt and for treating me like a real person ever since I was young. Thank you for taking me to Bluestockings, to Buvette, and, yes, even to see your life when I was small. (I mean it!) Thank you for being one of the most fascinating and astute conversationalists I know, even if you don't believe me, and for helping me wade through one of the hardest years of my life.

To Susan Lent: voice of Squirrely, curser/laugher extraordinaire, mom. Thank you for birthing me, of course—but you know I thank you for that every year. Really, thank you for supporting everything I pursue without ever seeming to doubt it, or me, for a second. I'm realizing more and more how rare that is. And I know you're proud of me when I do my own thing, but I owe it to you, at least in part, for raising me with the idea that a cookie-cutter path is just about the silliest thing you could follow if you don't want to be any old cookie. Thank you for being my mama. Love ya.

To everyone on both sides of my family. Thank you for your difficult history and your hilarity and your Passover pep talks and your warmth. Thank you for sending loving voicemails from the other side of the country and for opening your home to me even before we knew each other. And thank you to everyone who isn't here to see this part.

To Vera/Babs Zeldovich, Veebz, Doctor-Doctor vbz2, you. Thank you for being my fellow field mouse in the kitchen and my favorite companion to that overrated water park. Thank you for being an unimaginably important part of everything. What can I even write here? Well, picture a postcard on which I've described just how thoughtful and caring and unbelievably attuned to things you are, but on which that little barcode from the post office gets stamped at the bottom. Now you can no longer make out the crucial last row of letters— which, *phew*, because I don't know how exactly to describe how big a deal you are to me. Thank you for getting me through the past few years. And in case you missed it: I'm mega proud of you.

To Simon Lawrence, sL: there are no words, and I'm getting all tear-salted just writing this much. Thank you for being a preposterously splendid part of the universe, and of this book, and of this Lent. I don't know how I could have done this without you, or how to capture what you mean to me. You can imagine the number of times I've tried to write this, then decided that it didn't do you justice, then deleted and rewrote it, then deleted and rewrote it again. (Yeahhh, it's a good thing you didn't have to witness that part.) Thank you for every minute together. For that time you offered to get on the next train to DC, which time I think of often, but which is such an everyday part of your goodness that you probably don't even consider it a thing. Perhaps you're embarrassed to see said goodness spilled out all over this book—no longer a draft you're reading in the living room we shared, with that instinctive editing eye of yours, but in something printed and bound. Well, it's all still true. Thank you for the happiest times. For the hardest times. For all the times you made up a song about the Internet or explored a new place with me. Thank you for your generosity in the way that you love and for the fact that you're one of the only humans I would ever use that word for in earnest. How can I describe something—someone—epic without sounding cheesy? Thank you for being a Simon: not just past tense, but present and future.

To all my friends and family and acquaintances and writing buddies not named here: thank you for your fun and your thoughtfulness and your steadfastness and your writerly talks and your kind and good ideas. And to all the people I've met the past few years, or even once had a thought-provoking conversation with on the train: you're in here too.

# NOTES

**PART 1: COULD SOMEONE LOVE THIS BODY OF MINE**

1. Meridith Burles and Roanne Thomas, "'But They're Happening to You at the Wrong Time': Exploring Young Adult Women's Reflections on Serious Illness Through Photovoice," *Qualitative Social Work* 12, no. 5 (2012): 671–688, doi:10.1177/1473325012450484. There are few studies about young women's experiences with serious health issues, and some, like this one, are qualitative, meaning they present more feelings-oriented, descriptive results, rather than quantitative ones. (Some studies, however, do attempt to quantify feelings.) Many of these studies also have a small number of participants. But even when research has many participants and is more quantifiable, there's a critical discussion going on right now about which studies are valid or can be replicated. On top of that, scientific and health research has vastly overlooked several groups, including young women, women of color, trans women, and women in general. For this reason, I've included some of the studies that have been published, with the caveat that research has a long way to go. For expert thoughts on this enormous oversight in research on women, see part 4.

2. A paragraph in Christina Crosby, *A Body, Undone: Living On After Great Pain* (New York: New York University Press, 2016), helped crystalize this tension for me. As Crosby, an athletic professor whose bicycle accident caused her to become paralyzed from the breastbone down, writes, "Disability is created by building codes and education policy, subway elevators that don't work and school buses that don't arrive, and all the marginalization, exploitation, demeaning acts, and active exclusions that deny full access and equality to 'the disabled.' To focus on intractable pain, then, or grief at the loss of able-bodiedness, as I do here, may be thought to play into a pathologizing narrative that

would return disability to 'misshapen' bodies and 'abnormal' minds."
(That's the same pathologizing narrative that I don't want to feed
into.) Crosby nevertheless writes that for people whose lives are
"shaped by catastrophic accident," as hers is, or "chronic and progressive illness, or genetic predisposition," things like "pain and grief over
loss nonetheless remain as unavoidable facts."

3. David J. Tunnicliffe et al., "'Lupus Means Sacrifices': The Perspectives
of Adolescents and Young Adults with Systemic Lupus Erythematosus," *Arthritis Care & Research* 68, no. 6 (2016): 828–37, https://
ses.library.usyd.edu.au/bitstream/2123/15386/2/SLE_qualitative
_manuscript_040915_Tunnicliffe%20-%20Clean.pdf.

4. R. Odo and C. Potter, "Understanding the Needs of Young Adult Cancer Survivors: A Clinical Perspective," *Oncology (Williston Park)* 23
(October 2009): 23–27, www.ncbi.nlm.nih.gov/pubmed/19856605.

5. For instance, see Lois Romano, "Newt Gingrich, Maverick on the
Hill," *Washington Post*, January 3, 1985, https://www.washingtonpost
.com/archive/lifestyle/1985/01/03/newt-gingrich-maverick-on-the-hill
/46aab64f-7752-493d-b28b-9b675c0775b5/?utm_term=.83e3d1117099.
While some outlets (including the *Post*) have later published quotes
from Gingrich's daughters and others saying that the details in the account weren't fully accurate, still others have maintained that it was
accurate (and have questioned the move to discount it). The story, either way, is embedded in many people's memories.

6. Brian Ross and Rhonda Schwartz, "Exclusive: Gingrich Lacks Moral
Character to Be President, Ex-Wife Says," *ABC News*, January 19,
2012, http://abcnews.go.com/Blotter/exclusive-gingrich-lacks-moral
-character-president-wife/story?id=15392899.

7. Christine Hauser, "Padma Lakshmi Opens Up About Rushdie in Memoir," *New York Times*, March 9, 2016, https://www.nytimes.com/2016
/03/10/arts/padma-lakshmi-opens-up-about-rushdie-in-memoir.html.

8. Robert H. Carlson, "Study: Women with Brain Tumors Have 10 Times
Rate of Divorce as Men with Brain Tumors," *Oncology Times* 23, no. 8
(August 2001): 63, http://journals.lww.com/oncology-times/Fulltext
/2001/08000/Study__Women_with_Brain_Tumors_Have_10_Times
_Rate.24.aspx.

9. Ibid.

10. "Marriage More Likely to End in Divorce When Wives Get Sick, According to ISU Study," Iowa State University News Service, March 4,
2015, http://www.news.iastate.edu/news/2015/03/04/illnessdivorce.

11. Amelia Karraker and Kenzie Latham, "In Sickness and in Health?
Physical Illness as a Risk Factor for Marital Dissolution in Later Life,"
*Journal of Health and Social Behavior* 56 (2015): 420–35. This study,
inadvertently, provides an example of why we should take studies with

a grain of salt. The study I first found by Karraker and Latham was published in March 2015. When, in 2017, I later went to fact-check what I'd written down, I found that the March study had been retracted due to an error in the code used to analyze the findings and that a new version of the study—the one cited here—had been published in September 2015. It still showed that the onset of certain types of illness in a woman was associated with divorce, but the findings were somewhat toned down. For further explanation, see also Shannon Palus, "'To Our Horror': Widely Reported Study Suggesting Divorce Is More Likely When Wives Fall Ill Gets Axed," July 21, 2015, *Retraction Watch*, http://retractionwatch.com/2015/07/21/to-our -horror-widely-reported-study-suggesting-divorce-is-more-likely-when -wives-fall-ill-gets-axed. For the authors' own explanation for the retraction, see Amelia Karraker and Kenzie Latham, "Authors' Explanation of the Retraction," *Journal of Health and Social Behavior* 56, no. 3 (2015): 412–19, http://journals.sagepub.com/doi/pdf/10.1177 /0022146515595817.

12. Tara Parker-Pope, "Divorce Risk Higher When Wife Gets Sick," *New York Times*, November 12, 2009, https://well.blogs.nytimes.com/2009 /11/12/men-more-likely-to-leave-spouse-with-cancer; and Michael J. Glantz et al., "Gender Disparity in the Rate of Partner Abandonment in Patients with Serious Medical Illness," *Cancer* 115 (July 30, 2009), http://onlinelibrary.wiley.com/doi/10.1002/cncr.24577/full. See also Meredith Bryan, "Why Are These Men Leaving Their Wives?," *O, The Oprah Magazine*, August 2011, http://www.oprah.com/relationships /why-men-leave-sick-wives-facing-illness-alone-couples-and-cancer.

13. Cynthia A. Berg and Renn Upchurch, "A Developmental-Contextual Model of Couples Coping with Chronic Illness Across the Adult Life Span," *Psychological Bulletin* 133, no. 6 (2007): 920–54, https:// brainmass.com/file/344464/illness-adult+life+span.pdf, doi:10.1037 /0033-2909.133.6.920.

14. The so-called ugly laws, as Elizabeth Greiwe explains in the *Chicago Tribune*, were ordinances that cities across the country passed starting in 1867 in San Francisco (Elizabeth Greiwe, "Flashback: How an 'Ugly Law' Stayed on Chicago's Books for 93 Years," *Chicago Tribune*, June 23, 2016, http://www.chicagotribune.com/news/opinion/commentary /ct-ugly-laws-disabilities-chicago-history-flashback-perspec-0626-md -20160622-story.html). Chicago's own "ugly law," Greiwe writes, "banned anyone who was 'diseased, maimed, mutilated, or in any way deformed, so as to be an unsightly or disgusting object' from being in the 'public view.'" The Chicago city council didn't repeal the ordinance until 1974. See also Susan M. Schweik, *The Ugly Laws: Disability in Public* (New York: New York University Press, 2009).

15. A shout-out to Sandra Beasley, the poet and writer whose book *Don't Kill the Birthday Girl: Tales from an Allergic Life* (New York: Crown, 2011) includes the story of a date that ends in a dangerous food-allergy reaction after Beasley pretended to be fine during a meal.

16. Lisa Glatt, "The Atheist's Table," *Rattle* (blog), issue 25 (spring 2006), http://www.rattle.com/the-atheists-tunnel-by-lisa-glatt.

17. Adina Talve-Goodman, "I Must Have Been That Man," *Bellevue Literary Review* 15, no. 1 (spring 2015): 22.

18. This came up a lot in my research. But I also want to give credit to an essay that has always stuck with me: Sarah Manguso, "The Cure," *New York Times*, April 13, 2008. It's an excerpt from her memoir, *The Two Kinds of Decay* (New York: Farrar, Straus and Giroux, 2008). Manguso feels unattractive while going through major life-threatening health issues in college and while her body morphs into something she considers ugly because of the steroids she is on and her catheter scars. She attributes her recovery from illness to a friend's "selflessly" having sex with her.

19. Bella DePaulo, "Everything You Think You Know About Single People Is Wrong," *Washington Post*, February 8, 2016, https://www.washingtonpost.com/news/in-theory/wp/2016/02/08/everything-you-think-you-know-about-single-people-is-wrong/?utm_term=.d4d6eodbdb28.

20. Debbie Kralik, Tina Koch, and Sue Eastwood, "The Salience of the Body: Transition in Sexual Self-Identity for Women Living with Multiple Sclerosis," *Journal of Advanced Nursing* 42, no. 1 (2003): 11–20, doi:10.1046/j.1365–2648.2003.02505.x.

21. Talve-Goodman, "I Must Have Been That Man," 25.

22. Hiding comes up frequently. For another example, see Emily V. Gordon, "A Timeline of One Girl's Relationship with Her Body," *xojane*, April 26, 2012, http://www.xojane.com/healthy/timeline-girls-relationship-her-body, in which she hides being sick from her boyfriend until the point at which she's hospitalized for a month and needs to go on a ventilator to survive, which she does, but barely. And yet, she says, "old habits die hard." During her first episode of the disease since the hospital stay, she hides it from him again.

23. Julie Beck, "New Research Says There Are Only Four Emotions," Atlantic.com, February 4, 2014, https://www.theatlantic.com/health/archive/2014/02/new-research-says-there-are-only-four-emotions/283560.

24. For instance, see Arnaud Leleu et al., "The Odor Context Facilitates the Perception of Low-Intensity Facial Expressions of Emotion," *PLoS ONE* 10, no. 9 (2015): e0138656, doi:10.1371/journal.pone.0138656.

25. Anne Thomas, "Dating in a Wheelchair: Your Problem, Not Mine," Women in the World series, *New York Times*, April 8, 2015, http://

nytlive.nytimes.com/womenintheworld/2015/04/08/dating-in-a
-wheelchair-your-problem-not-mine.

26. Samantha Irby, "I Wore a Diaper to Speed Dating," *Bitches Gotta Eat* (blog), January 10, 2011, http://bitchesgottaeat.blogspot.com/2011/01 /i-wore-diaper-to-speed-dating.html.

27. Samantha Irby, "The Trouble with Getting Married When You Are Already Old," *Bitches Gotta Eat* (blog), June 17, 2016, http://bitchesgotta eat.blogspot.com/2016/06/the-trouble-with-getting-married-when.html.

28. Aside from the books mentioned here, see, for example, Public Affairs, UC Berkeley, "Top Disability Scholar Leaving Yale for Berkeley," November 17, 2015, *Berkeley News*, http://news.berkeley.edu/2015/11/17 /top-disability-scholar-leaving-yale-for-berkeley. See also "Disability Studies and LGBTQ Issues" in *Proud Heritage: People, Issues, and Documents of the LGBT Experience*, ed. Chuck Stewart (Santa Barbara, CA: ABC-CLIO, 2015), 141, and essays such as "The Queer Life of Chronic Pain," *Dazed*, accessed June 1, 2017, a wonderful piece by Brittany Newell, http://www.dazeddigital.com/artsandculture/article/35151 /1/the-queer-life-of-chronic-pain-brittany-newell.

29. Carolyn Yates, "Poly Pocket: Being as Direct as Possible," *Autostraddle*, November 17, 2016, https://www.autostraddle.com/poly-pocket -being-as-direct-as-possible-358566.

30. Gwyneth Ferguson Matthews, *Voices from the Shadows: Women with Disabilities Speak Out* (Toronto: Women's Press, 1983), 62.

31. Audre Lorde, *The Cancer Journals*, special ed. (San Francisco: Aunt Lute Books, 1997), 57.

32. Christina Cooke, "To Save African Penguins, Humans Set Up a Dating Service," *New York Times*, November 23, 2015, https://www.nytimes .com/2015/11/24/science/to-save-african-penguins-humans-run-a -dating-service.html.

33. Sandra Beasley, *Don't Kill the Birthday Girl: Tales from an Allergic Life* (New York: Broadway Paperbacks/Crown/Random House, 2011), 11, Google Books edition.

**PART 2: THE (FOGGY) GLASS CEILING AND THE WALL**

1. P. A. Gordon, M. Stoelb, and J. Chiriboga, "The Vocational Implication of Two Common Rheumatic Diseases," *Journal of Rehabilitation* 63, no. 1 (January–March 1997), https://www.questia.com/library /journal/1G1-19178149/the-vocational-implication-of-two-common -rheumatic.

2. Reshma Jagsi et al., "Impact of Adjuvant Chemotherapy on Long-Term Employment of Survivors of Early-Stage Breast Cancer," *Cancer* 120, no. 12 (June 2014): 1854–1862, doi:10.1002/cncr.28607.

3. Caryl Rivers and Rosalind C. Barnett, *The New Soft War on Women: How the Myth of Female Ascendance Is Hurting Women, Men—and Our Economy* (New York: Jeremy P. Tarcher/Penguin, 2013), Google Books edition.

4. Katherine Russell Rich, "A Mass for Katherine," *Washington Post*, July 9, 2000, https://www.washingtonpost.com/archive/lifestyle/2000/07/09/a-mass-for-katherine/2dea2fb4-95d0-4124-8fd0-ea962818bb52/?utm_term=.71b85f6cc497.

5. Margalit Fox, "Katherine Russell Rich, Who Wrote of Battle with Cancer, Dies at 56," *New York Times*, April 6, 2012, http://www.nytimes.com/2012/04/07/health/katherine-russell-rich-who-wrote-of-cancer-fight-dies-at-56.html.

6. Esmé Weijun Wang, "I'm Chronically Ill and Afraid of Being Lazy," *Elle.com*, April 26, 2016, http://www.elle.com/life-love/a35930/chronically-ill-afraid-lazy.

7. Samantha Kittle, "Friday Night. No Plans," *A Lie of the Mind* (blog), 2014, http://www.alieofthemind.com/post/75212348146/friday-night-no-plans-there-are-few-steps-in.

8. "Equal Pay & the Wage Gap," National Women's Law Center, https://nwlc.org/issue/equal-pay-and-the-wage-gap.

9. "The Lifetime Wage Gap, State by State," National Women's Law Center, https://nwlc.org/resources/the-lifetime-wage-gap-state-by-state.

10. Kevin Miller, "The Simple Truth about the Gender Pay Gap," spring 2017, American Association of University Women, http://www.aauw.org/research/the-simple-truth-about-the-gender-pay-gap.

**PART 3: IT'S COOL GUYS I'M TOTALLY FINE**

1. Amy Berkowitz, *Tender Points* (Oakland, CA: Timeless, Infinite Light, 2015), 43.

2. Michael Bury, "Chronic Illness as Biographical Disruption," *Sociology of Health & Illness* 4, no. 2 (1982): 167–82, doi:10.1111/1467-9566.ep11339939.

3. Elizabeth J. Susman, Lorah D. Dorn, and Virginia L. Schiefelbein, "Puberty, Sexuality, and Health," in *Handbook of Psychology*, vol. 6, *Developmental Psychology*, ed. Richard M. Lerner, M. Ann Easterbrooks, and Jayanthi Mistry (Hoboken, NJ: Wiley, 2003), 305, Google Books edition.

4. Rosanna M. Bertrand and Margie E. Lachman, "Personality Development in Adulthood and Old Age," in *Handbook of Psychology*, vol. 6, *Developmental Psychology*, ed. Richard M. Lerner, M. Ann Easterbrooks, and Jayanthi Mistry (Hoboken, NJ: Wiley, 2003), 473, Google Books edition.

5. Samantha Irby, "Potty Mouth," *Bitches Gotta Eat* (blog), July 22, 2010, http://bitchesgottaeat.blogspot.com/2010/07/potty-mouth.html.

6. Ibid.

7. Samantha Kittle, "You're Gonna Like the Way You Look. I Guarantee It," *A Lie of the Mind* (blog), http://www.alieofthemind.com/page/15, accessed June 1, 2017.

8. Lorde, *The Cancer Journals*, 11.

9. Matthews, *Voices from the Shadows*, 23.

10. Irby, "I Wore a Diaper to Speed Dating."

11. Suleika Jaouad, "Life, Interrupted: Facing Cancer in Your 20s," *New York Times*, March 29, 2012, https://well.blogs.nytimes.com/2012/03/29/life-interrupted-facing-cancer-in-your-20s.

12. Deborah Orr, "10 Things Not to Say to Someone When They're Ill," *Guardian*, April 18, 2012, https://www.theguardian.com/lifeandstyle/2012/apr/18/10-things-not-say-when-ill.

13. Emily McDowell, "Empathy Cards for Serious Illness," *Things & Stuff* (blog of Emily McDowell Studio), May 3, 2015, https://emilymcdowell.com/blogs/all/105537926-empathy-cards-for-serious-illness.

14. "Empathy™: What to Say, When You Don't Know What to Say," Emily McDowell Studio, https://emilymcdowell.com/collections/empathy-cards, accessed June 1, 2017.

15. McDowell, "Empathy Cards for Serious Illness."

16. Heather Ashley, "Why I Feel More Comfortable with Older People as a Young Woman with Chronic Illness," *The Mighty* (blog), December 15, 2016, https://themighty.com/2016/12/being-friends-with-older-people-while-sick.

17. National Institute of Allergy and Infectious Disease, "Gender-Specific Health Challenges Facing Women," National Institutes of Health, National Institute of Allergy and Infectious Disease, last updated July 14, 2016, https://www.niaid.nih.gov/research/gender-specific-health-challenges.

18. Stupid Cancer, "About Us," www.stupidcancer.org/about.

19. First Descents, www.firstdescents.org; Samfund, www.thesamfund.org; Young Survival Coalition, www.youngsurvival.org; Lacuna Loft, www.lacunaloft.org.

20. "Who Gets Lupus," Lupus Research Alliance, http://www.lupusny.org/about-lupus/who-gets-lupus, accessed June 1, 2017.

21. "African American Women Develop Lupus at a Younger Age," Emory News Center, Emory University, October 28, 2013, http://news.emory.edu/stories/2013/10/lupus_and_african_american_women/campus.html.

22. S. Sam Lim et al., "The Incidence and Prevalence of Systemic Lupus Erythematosus, 2002–2004: The Georgia Lupus Registry," *Arthritis & Rheumatology* 66 (2014): 357–68, doi:10.1002/art.38239.

23. Joan Jacobs Brumberg, *The Body Project: An Intimate History of American Girls* (New York: Random House, 1998), 107.

24. Meridith Bland, "The Saturday Rumpus Essay: All Bodies Count," *Rumpus*, April 18, 2015, http://therumpus.net/2015/04/the-saturday-rumpus-essay-all-bodies-count.

25. Wolfgang Linden et al., "Anxiety and Depression After Cancer Diagnosis: Prevalence Rates by Cancer Type, Gender, and Age," *Journal of Affective Disorders* 141, no. 2 (2012): 343–51, doi:10.1016/j.jad.2012.03.025.

**PART 4: WHY DON'T THEY BELIEVE ME?**

1. Examples of doctors' failure or refusal to believe women are more numerous than I can squeeze into one section. The legacy of "hysteria," now sometimes called *conversion disorder*, still haunts the perception of women who present with symptoms that doctors can't immediately trace. This history, which many have written about, dates back millennia and includes the idea, from Ancient Greece, that the uterus had been "poisoned by venomous humors, due to a lack of orgasms" (see C. Tasca et al., "Women and Hysteria in the History of Mental Health," *Clinical Practice & Epidemiology in Mental Health* 8 (2012): 110–19, https://www.ncbi.nlm.nih.gov/pmc/articles/PMC3480686). For a few examples: One fifteen-year-old young woman with lupus told researchers, "I mean GPs do have to understand a lot of different diseases. Perhaps he wasn't a great GP [general practitioner, or primary care physician] and couldn't put my symptoms together. I was kind of unhappy with that, not being taken seriously. I guess I kind of doubted if I was sick, I thought I was kind of imagining these things. Like am I doing it for attention? Am I crazy?" (Tunnicliffe et al., "Lupus Means Sacrifices"). See also Jennifer Brea's examples, a few paragraphs later in the text.

2. Kelly M. Hoffman, Sophie Trawalter, Jordan R. Axt, and M. Norman Oliver, "Racial Bias in Pain Assessment and Treatment Recommendations, and False Beliefs About Biological Differences Between Blacks and Whites," *Proceedings of National Academy of Sciences* 113, no. 16 (2016): 4296–301, http://m.pnas.org/content/113/16/4296.full.

3. Barbara Ehrenreich and Deirdre English, *Complaints & Disorders: The Sexual Politics of Sickness*, 2nd ed. (New York: Feminist Press, 2011): 41.

4. Ibid., 43.

5. Hoffman et al., "Racial Bias in Pain Assessment."

6. Diane E. Hoffmann and Anita J. Tarzian, "The Girl Who Cried Pain: A Bias Against Women in the Treatment of Pain," *Journal of Law, Medicine & Ethics* 29 (2001): 13–27, quoted in Joe Fassler, "How Doctors

Take Women's Pain Less Seriously," *Atlantic*, which in turn found the Hoffmann and Tarzian paper through Leslie Jamison's well-known essay, "Grand Unified Theory of Female Pain," *VQR, A National Journal of Literature & Discussion*, spring 2014, http://www.vqronline.org /essays-articles/2014/04/grand-unified-theory-female-pain.

7. Jennifer Brea, "What Happens When You Have a Disease Doctors Can't Diagnose," talk at TED Summit, June 2016, TED video, 17:07, https://www.ted.com/talks/jen_brea_what_happens_when_you_have_a _disease_doctors_can_t_diagnose.

8. Matthews, *Voices from the Shadows*, 83

9. For instance, see Philip Bump, "Study: Cops Tend to See Black Kids as Less Innocent than White Kids," Atlantic.com, March 10, 2014, https://www.theatlantic.com/national/archive/2014/03/cops-tend-to-see -black-kids-as-less-innocent-than-white-kids/383247.

10. Jen Chung, "Second Patient Says Mt. Sinai Doctor Sexually Abused Her," *Gothamist*, January 20, 2016, http://gothamist.com/2016/01/20 /mt_sinai_doctor_sex_assault.php.

11. A shout-out to documentary filmmaker Maggie Hadleigh-West, who got me thinking about the continuum of sexual harassment and sexual assault at a screening of her street-harassment film *War Zone*.

12. Patricia Harman, *The Blue Cotton Gown: A Midwife's Memoir* (Boston: Beacon Press, 2008), 105–9.

13. Carrie Teegardin, Danny Robbins, Jeff Ernsthausen, and Ariel Hart, "License to Betray: A Broken System Forgives Sexually Abusive Doctors in Every State, Investigation Finds," part 1 of Doctors & Sex Abuse series, *Atlanta Journal-Constitution*, July 6, 2016, http://doctors .ajc.com/doctors_sex_abuse/?ecmp=doctorssexabuse_microsite_nav.

14. Ariel Hart, "Which Doctors Are Sexually Abusive?" Doctors & Sex Abuse series, *Atlanta Journal-Constitution*, 2016, http://doctors.ajc .com/doctors_who_sexually_abuse/?ecmp=doctorssexabuse_microsite _stories.

15. Jeff Ernsthausen, "Fact-Checking the Data Bank System," Doctors & Sexual Abuse series, *Atlanta Journal-Constitution*, July 6, 2016, http:// doctors.ajc.com/database_explainer.

16. Jaime M. Grant et al., *National Transgender Discrimination Survey Report on Health and Health Care* (Washington, DC: National Center for Transgender Equality/National Gay and Lesbian Task Force, October 2010), http://www.thetaskforce.org/static_html/downloads /resources_and_tools/ntds_report_on_health.pdf.

17. Sandy E. James et al., *The Report of the 2015 U.S. Transgender Survey* (Washington, DC: National Center for Transgender Equality, December 2016), http://www.transequality.org/sites/default/files/docs/usts /USTS%20Full%20Report%20%20FINAL%201.6.17.pdf.

18. Ibid.

19. *Transgender-Affirming Hospital Policies: Creating Equal Access to Quality Health Care for Transgender Patients*, Human Rights Campaign, Lambda Legal, and the LGBTQ Rights Committee of the New York City Bar Association, revised May 2016, http://www.hrc.org /resources/transgender-affirming-hospital-policies.

20. Lorde, *The Cancer Journals*, 57.

21. Ibid, 58, 60. Here, Lorde also recounts how the doctor's nurse, "in the offices of one of the top breast cancer surgeons in New York City," told her that they would like Lorde to wear a prosthesis, as otherwise her appearance would be "bad for the morale of the office."

22. Office of Disease Prevention and Health Promotion, "Lesbian, Gay, Bisexual, and Transgender Health," HealthyPeople.gov, https://www .healthypeople.gov/2020/topics-objectives/topic/lesbian-gay-bisexual -and-transgender-health?topicid=25, accessed June 1, 2017.

23. Roni Caryn Rabin, "'Going Flat' After Breast Cancer," *New York Times*, October 31, 2016, https://www.nytimes.com/2016/11/01/well /live/going-flat-after-breast-cancer.html?_r=0.

24. National Institute of Allergy and Infectious Disease, "Gender-Specific Health Challenges Facing Women."

25. Martha E. Banks and Ellyn Kaschak, *Women with Visible and Invisible Disabilities: Multiple Intersections, Multiple Issues, Multiple Therapies* (New York: Routledge, 2013), xxiv, Google Books edition.

26. M. B. Yunus, "Gender Differences in Fibromyalgia and Other Related Syndromes," *Journal of Gender-Specific Medicine* 5, no. 2 (2002): 42–47, https://www.ncbi.nlm.nih.gov/pubmed/11974674.

27. Anne Werner, Lise Widding Isaksen, and Kirsti Malterud, "'I Am Not the Kind of Woman Who Complains of Everything': Illness Stories on Self and Shame in Women with Chronic Pain," *Social Science & Medicine* 59, no. 5 (2004): 1035–1045, doi:10.1016/j.socscimed .2003.12.001.

28. Miriam E. Tucker, "With His Son Terribly Ill, a Top Scientist Takes on Chronic Fatigue Syndrome," *Washington Post*, October 5, 2015, https:// www.washingtonpost.com/national/health-science/with-his-son-terribly -ill-a-top-scientist-takes-on-chronic-fatigue-syndrome/2015/10/05 /c5d6189c-4041-11e5-8d45-d815146f81fa_story.html.

29. Pavel V. Ovseiko et al., "A Global Call for Action to Include Gender in Research Impact Assessment," *Health Research Policy and Systems* 14, no. 50 (2016), doi: 10.1186/s12961-016-0126-z.

30. Julie Rovner, "GAO: NIH Needs to Do More to Ensure Research Evaluates Gender Differences," *Washington Post*, November 28, 2015, https://www.washingtonpost.com/national/health-science/gao-nih-needs -to-do-more-to-ensure-research-evaluates-gender-differences/2015

/11/28/902ed502-9524-11e5-8aa0-5d0946560a97_story.html?utm
_term=.fc5c8141d413.

31. Ibid.

32. "PrEP," Centers for Disease Control and Prevention, last updated April 17, 2017, https://www.cdc.gov/hiv/basics/prep.html.

33. Katie Hail-Jares et al., "Knowledge Is Power: PrEP, TasP, and Healthcare Access Among DC Street-Based Sex Workers," 2016, academic poster provided by Hail-Jares via e-mail.

34. Ibid.

35. "Facts About the Over-Incarceration of Women in the United States," American Civil Liberties Union, https://www.aclu.org/other/facts-about -over-incarceration-women-united-states; and "Statistics on Women Offenders—2015," Court Services and Offender Supervision Agency for the District of Columbia, http://www.csosa.gov/reentry/news /statistics-on-women-offenders-2015.pdf, accessed June 1, 2017.

36. Patricia A. Kaufert, "Screening the Body: The Pap Smear and the Mammogram," in *Living and Working with the New Medical Technologies: Intersections of Inquiry*, ed. Margaret Lock, Allan Young, and Alberto Cambrosio (New York: Cambridge University Press, 2000), 167.

### PART 5: TO RAISE SMALL HUMANS—OR NOT

1. Tunnicliffe et al., "Lupus Means Sacrifices."

2. Reniqua Allen, "Is Egg Freezing Only for White Women?," *New York Times*, May 21, 2016, https://www.nytimes.com/2016/05/22/opinion /is-egg-freezing-only-for-white-women.html.

3. Elizabeth A. Stewart et al., "The Burden of Uterine Fibroids for African-American Women: Results of a National Survey," *Journal of Women's Health* 22, no. 10 (2013): 807–816, https://www.ncbi.nlm.nih.gov/pmc /articles/PMC3787340; and Vanessa L. Jacoby et al., "Racial and Ethnic Disparities in Benign Gynecologic Conditions and Associated Surgeries," *American Journal of Obstetrics and Gynecology* 202, no. 6 (2010): 514–521, https://www.ncbi.nlm.nih.gov/pmc/articles/PMC4625911.

4. Margarett Shnorhavorian et al., "Fertility Preservation Knowledge, Counseling, and Actions Among Adolescent and Young Adult Cancer Patients: A Population-Based Study," *Cancer* 121, no. 19 (2015): 3499–506, https://www.ncbi.nlm.nih.gov/pmc/articles/PMC4734641/.

5. See, for example, "Dampened Immunity During Pregnancy Promotes Evolution of More Virulent Flu," *Science Daily*, March 8 2017, https:// www.sciencedaily.com/releases/2017/03/170308145347.htm.

6. Anyesuki, "I Would Rather Have Lupus than Children," comment on Reddit, January 9, 2015, https://www.reddit.com/r/childfree /comments/2rwqhv/i_would_rather_have_lupus_than_children /#bottom-comments.

7. Although there are guidelines for preventing transmission of HIV during childbirth, there are still risks. According to NIH, babies are tested after they're born to make sure that the precautions worked, and there is a set of guidelines if the baby does indeed test positive. In addition, some women give birth vaginally and others by C-section, depending on various risk factors. See US Department of Health and Human Services, "HIV and Pregnancy: Preventing Mother-to-Child Transmission of HIV After Birth," *AIDSinfo*, November 14, 2016, https://aidsinfo.nih.gov/education-materials/fact-sheets/24/71/preventing -mother-to-child-transmission-of-hiv-after-birth; and US Department of Health and Human Services, "HIV and Pregnancy: HIV Medicines During Pregnancy and Childbirth," *AIDSinfo*, November 14, 2016, https://aidsinfo.nih.gov/education-materials/fact-sheets/24/70/hiv -medicines-during-pregnancy-and-childbirth.

8. Matthews, *Voices from the Shadows*, 98–99.

### PART 6: SICK LIKE MISS AMERICA

1. Blain Roberts, "The Miss America Pageant Stills Sends the Wrong Message," Room for Debate, *New York Times*, September 12, 2013, http://www.nytimes.com/roomfordebate/2013/09/12/is-the-miss-america -pageant-bad-for-women/the-miss-america-pageant-stills-sends-the -wrong-message.

2. Lisa Marsh, "Your New Miss America Might Be Beautiful—and Bald," Today.com, January 11, 2011, http://www.today.com/style/your-new -miss-america-might-be-beautiful-bald-wbna41021492.

3. Miriam E. Tucker, "Hey, Miss Idaho, Is That an Insulin Pump on Your Bikini?" NPR.org, July 17, 2014, http://www.npr.org/sections/health -shots/2014/07/17/332255209/hey-miss-idaho-is-that-an-insulin-pump -on-your-bikini. Tucker writes that she herself wears an insulin pump, so she is reporting on Miss Idaho's appearance from a place of first-hand experience. See also Greta VanDyke, "Miss Idaho Gives Type 1 Diabetics Brave Role Model," *Idaho Press-Tribune*, November 4, 2014, http://www.idahopress.com/members/miss-idaho-gives-type -diabetics-brave-role-model/article_549a6e2a-63d4-11e4-93a4 -278a8e48b0a5.html; and Tara Fowler, "Miss Idaho Sierra Sanderson [*sic*] Wears Insulin Pump on Stage," People.com, July 18, 2014, http://people.com/celebrity/miss-idaho-sierra-sanderson-wears-insulin-pump -on-stage.

4. Sierra Sandison, "Defeating Diabetes," Miss Idaho Organization, July 15, 2014, http://www.missidaho.org/blog/2014/07/wow-wow-wow -where-do-i-even-start-i.html.

5. "Colostomy Bag Bikini Photograph Seen by Nine Million," *BBC News*, July 3, 2014, http://www.bbc.com/news/uk-england-hereford-worcester

-28138482; K. C. Blumm, "Former Model Poses in Bikini with Colostomy Bags," *People*, July 2, 2014, http://people.com/celebrity/former-model-bethany-townsend-poses-in-bikini-with-colostomy-bags; Scott Stump, "'I Wasn't Ashamed': Woman with Crohn's Disease Shows Off Colostomy Bags in Stunning Photo," Today.com, July 3, 2014, http://www.today.com/health/crohns-disease-sufferer-shows-colostomy-bags-stunning-photo-1D79884421; Eleanor Goldberg, "Aspiring Model with Crohn's Disease Isn't Afraid to Show Colostomy Bags in Bikini Photo," *Huffington Post*, July 1, 2014, http://www.huffingtonpost.com/2014/07/01/colostomy-bag-model-picture_n_5548863.html; Eleanor Goldberg, "Another Model Proves You Can Be a Sexy Centerfold While Revealing Colostomy Bags," *Huffington Post*, August 1, 2014, http://www.huffingtonpost.com/2014/08/01/male-model-colostomy-bags_n_5639347.html.

6. Caters News, "Stunning Brunette Bravely Posts First-Ever Bikini Picture Exposing Her Colostomy Bags," *New York Daily News*, July 2, 2014, http://www.nydailynews.com/life-style/health/woman-posts-bikini-pic-exposing-colostomy-bags-article-1.1852000; Darcie Loreno, "Bombshell Bears All, Shows Colostomy Bag to the World to Make an Important Point," *Fox 8 Cleveland*, July 3, 2014, http://fox8.com/2014/07/03/bombshell-bears-all-shows-colostomy-bag-to-the-world-to-make-an-important-point.

7. "The Telegraph's 100 Britons of the Year 2014," *Telegraph*, http://www.telegraph.co.uk/news/uknews/11304173/Telegraphs-Britons-of-the-year.html?frame=3147098.

8. Hannah Gale, "Model Who Went Viral with Colostomy Bag Pic Is Targeted for Being Too Skinny, Despite It Being Caused by Her Life-Threatening Illness," Metro.co.uk, July 7, 2014, http://metro.co.uk/2014/07/07/model-who-went-viral-for-colostomy-bag-pic-is-targeted-for-being-too-skinny-despite-it-being-caused-by-her-life-threatening-illness-4789327. See also this story by a teenage girl who has Graves' disease and is picked on for being "too thin," even though her thinness is caused by the disease: Emily Leon, "Being Thin Isn't All It's Cracked Up to Be, Teen Says," *Women's eNews*, May 18, 2016, http://womensenews.org/2016/05/being-thin-isnt-all-its-cracked-up-to-be-teen-says.

9. Irene McGee, "Slaps, Lies, and Videotape: Irene's True Story of 1998's *The Real World: Seattle*," *Vulture*, November 22, 2013, http://www.vulture.com/2013/11/real-world-seattle-irene-slap-her-story.html.

10. Judy Z. Segal, "The Sexualization of the Medical," *Journal of Sex Research* 49, no. 4 (2012): 369–78, doi:10.1080/00224499.2011.653608.

11. Harley Pasternak, "2 Inspiring Women Who Prove Beauty Is More Than Skin Deep," *People*, July 23, 2014, http://greatideas.people.com/2014/07/23/harley-pasternak-inspiring-women.

12. "Wanda Sykes Talks About Breast Cancer," *Ellen* (TV show), video, September 2011, posted September 23, 2011, http://www.ellentv.com /2011/09/26/wanda-sykes-talks-about-breast-cancer.

13. Katy Waldman, "Stop Demanding Positivity from Cancer Survivors," *Slate*, November 25, 2013, http://www.slate.com/blogs/xx_factor/2013 /11/25/depression_after_cancer_chemo_sucks_and_we_shouldn_t _expect_cancer_survivors.html.

14. Judy Z. Segal, "Cancer Experience and Its Narration: An Accidental Study," *Literature and Medicine* 30, no. 2 (2012): 292–318, doi:10.1353/lm.2012.0017.

15. Daniela Olszewska, "Thirteenz," *Birdfeast* 9, http://www.birdfeast magazine.com/issuenine/olszewska.html, accessed June 1, 2017.

16. Rich, "A Mass for Katherine."

17. Jason Zinoman, "Going Topless, Tig Notaro Takes Over Town Hall," *New York Times*, November 7, 2014, https://www.nytimes.com/2014 /11/08/arts/going-topless-tig-notaro-takes-over-town-hall.html.

18. "Sickness & Health," *Woman of the Hour, with Lena Dunham* (podcast series), season 2, episode 9, in *Lenny*, January 19, 2017, http:// www.lennyletter.com/culture/a697/women-of-the-hour-sickness -health-season-2-episode-9.

19. Melody Chiu, "Selena Gomez Taking Time Off After Dealing with 'Anxiety, Panic Attacks and Depression' Due to Her Lupus Diagnosis," People.com, August 30, 2016, http://people.com/celebrity/selena -gomez-taking-a-break-after-lupus-complications/.

20. Eliza Berman, "How *The Fault in Our Stars* Dramatically Improves the 'Sick Flick,'" *Slate*, June 5, 2014, http://www.slate.com/blogs /browbeat/2014/06/05/the_fault_in_our_stars_review_the_sick_flick _reinvented_with_shailene_woodley.html. See also Roger Ebert, "For Roseanna," *Rogerebert.com*, July 25, 1997, http://www.rogerebert .com/reviews/for-roseanna-1997, in which the original quote appears.

21. Ibid.

# INDEX